Gordon Parker is Scientia Professor of Psychiatry at the University of NSW, Professorial Fellow at the Black Dog Institute, and a renowned researcher and expert on mood disorders. **Kerrie Eyers** is a psychologist and Publications Consultant at the Black Dog Institute, Sydney. Gordon Parker and Kerrie Eyers are editors of the bestselling *Journeys with the Black Dog* and several other books on depression. **Philip Boyce** is Professor of Psychiatry at the University of Sydney, Professorial Fellow at the Black Dog Institute, and an international expert on postnatal depression.

Overcoming Baby Blues

A comprehensive guide to perinatal depression

GORDON PARKER,
KERRIE EYERS
and
PHILIP BOYCE

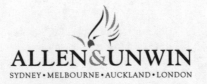

ALLEN&UNWIN
SYDNEY · MELBOURNE · AUCKLAND · LONDON

First published in 2014

Allen & Unwin
Sydney, Melbourne, Auckland, London

83 Alexander Street
Crows Nest NSW 2065
Australia
Phone: (61 2) 8425 0100
Email: info@allenandunwin.com
Web: www.allenandunwin.com

Cataloguing-in-Publication details are available
from the National Library of Australia
www.trove.nla.gov.au

ISBN 978 1 74331 677 1

Index by Puddingburn
Set in 12/15 pt Minion Pro by Midland Typesetters, Australia
Printed and bound in Australia by Griffin Press

10 9 8 7 6 5 4 3 2 1

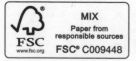

The paper in this book is FSC® certified.
FSC® promotes environmentally responsible,
socially beneficial and economically viable
management of the world's forests.

To Guy and Eve Sheppard

This book is dedicated to Guy and Eve Sheppard who supported the Black Dog Institute from its beginning. They spoke from the heart at the Institute's launch by Premier Bob Carr in 2002. Over the next decade they offered practical support in so many ways—including organising fundraising and fun-filled dinners—and always promoted the Institute's objectives of assisting better understanding and management of mood disorders.

Contents

List of tables and figures

Preface

Hope is like a road in the country: there was never a road, but when many people walk on it, the road comes into existence.

Lin Yutang

Mood problems following the birth of a baby (the period we refer to as *postnatal*) or before and after the birth (termed *perinatal*) are common, often debilitating and, frankly, unjust. We define these conditions, and the term perinatal, in Chapter 1.

During pregnancy many women experience depressive symptoms and approximately 10 per cent of those develop clinical depression. Following the birth, 60–80 per cent of mothers have the 'baby blues', while 10–15 per cent of women progress to a clinical mood disorder. By 'clinical' here, we mean that the disorder is severe, disabling and persistent, and likely to benefit from assessment and management by a health professional.

Being pregnant is tough enough without depression as well. After the celebration, usually, of a positive pregnancy test and the 'lock-in' emotional impact of the early baby pictures from the eight-week ultrasound, the pre-labour hard yards are yet to be run. Months of draining disruptions to sleep, as well as alterations to body shape and plumbing, are interwoven with rituals that mark pregnancy more as a rite of passage than a journey. Newer rituals such as boot-camp bonding with other mothers at antenatal classes, and older rituals such as the celebratory baby shower (preceding the whirlpool of birth) build to an ovation to celebrate the launching of a new human being into the world.

The hard labour of birth—together with the placing of a baby in the mother's arms—are expected to incite maternal euphoria and tribal jubilation. The woman has a new status—'mother'—and she is expected to be in a state of wonderment, exalted by the 'miracle of birth'. The baby—by its appearance, movement, snuggling and other instinctive strategies—is expected to activate immediate attachment links with the mother, while her facial responses in turn activate mirror neurons in the infant that begin to build the mother–child bond. But what if depression extinguishes the light in that new mother's eyes?

After such a long-distance race, mothers deserve to appreciate the wonders of their newborn, the joy and congratulations of family members and friends, and a guilt-free glass of champagne. To be hit with a mood disorder in the following days or months is painful enough, but going as it does against all the expectations associated with being a new mother, it is doubly hurtful. Depression and anxiety erode self-worth, confidence and ability to function. Warmth and congratulations from family and friends may make the struggling mother feel even more troubled. Through her darkened lens, she knows that unless she replies with 'I feel fine', she will be identified as failing. The emptiness and wasteland of her depression make her judge her responses as shallow at best and fake at worst. When she perceives her depression as compromising the bond with her child she feels shame as well. Despite depression having been largely destigmatised in recent decades, some of the most entrenched stigma still lies in the motherland of perinatal depression.

This book will take readers into the realm of perinatal mood disorders, and offer pointers for when intervention and management are needed. The good news is that these conditions are very responsive to treatment and support. For this reason, we argue for the importance of identifying the differing mood states, their causes and the management approaches most likely to bring benefit. This reflects the Black Dog Institute's longstanding model that depression is not an 'it' and that there should be no one-size-fits-all management model. Each sufferer experiences different mood conditions and each has their own narrative or personal story. Both components command respect and attention.

One mother made this appeal:

> *I would have liked my doctor to talk to me. To see me as an individual. To look up from my baby and ask how I was getting on. To listen for my particular circumstances, my experiences. To not lump me with general solutions that didn't apply to me, and too quickly, so that it became a one-size-fits-none experience.*

We will explain the main types of conditions that can occur during the perinatal period, and provide signals and early warning signs of each to sharpen your observations and understanding, and ideally assist your choice of management options.

Importantly, we wish to emphasise that, whatever the type of perinatal mood disorder, be it the blues at one end of the spectrum or the shocking experience of puerperal psychosis at the other, sufferers should expect and work towards a very optimistic outcome. Many perinatal problems dissipate spontaneously, while the few that persist benefit from professional intervention and targeted strategies. With this book we hope to assist you with decisions about when and how to seek intervention and who to turn to for professional help, thus moving beyond outcomes born of chance and guesswork. We trust that it will bring hope to those struggling with a mood disorder and assist in reducing the stigma experienced by these mothers who badly need their community's support. There is also a chapter for fathers and other family members, to help everyone navigate a path towards understanding and satisfaction. Note that throughout the book, when talking about couples, the use of 'he' and 'she' or 'mother' and 'father' is only for convenience. The information here is equally useful for couples of all persuasions.

Since 2007 we have published several books that build on the experiences of thousands of people who have contributed to the annual Black Dog Institute writing competitions by recounting their observations, hard-won wisdom and lessons learned—invariably with grit and sagacity, and often with wit and sharp insights. In this book, we act as editors of these stories, seeking to blend our essayists' views from the inside out with our clinical and research experience from the outside in. These differing perspectives complement each other and make it clear that without information from the sufferers themselves doctors and health professionals are working in the dark. It is important for everyone attempting to support sufferers of perinatal mood disorders to be aware of just how much they *are* suffering, and to move beyond factual awareness to an empathic understanding and a recognition that we are all in this together.

The entries in the 2011 'Postnatal Depression' Writing Competition gave us more than 200 essays to draw on here, and we have used pseudonyms to protect the privacy of those who have taken us into their world. Our essayists—including those quoted here—do not reflect the 'average' experience of the blues or the 'average' clinical depressive episode. Most women had experienced episodes so severe that they were brought to their knees by depression's horrors and its consequences—and yet they have moved on, overcoming the experience, and restoring and strengthening the sometimes disrupted relationship with their child.

You will feel these mothers' despair as they recount the bleakness of their world when they were depressed, and often the insensitivity of others … from friends who disappeared, to professionals who ranged from uncaring to punitive. But as these mothers' stories unfold, you will appreciate there is always hope. Sufferers should confidently expect that their postnatal mood disorder will vanish or be brought under control. And equally importantly, that in the process they will learn something about themselves and become more resilient to the stresses of modern life.

We thank the many people who have assisted the birth of this book—Guy and Eve Sheppard; Professor Helen Christensen, Executive Director of the Black Dog Institute; Dr Vered Gordon, the Institute's General Practice Program Developer; psychiatrists Professors Marie-Paule Austin and Bryanne Barnett; research assistants Amelia Paterson and Stacey McCraw; Dr Heather Brotchie; clinical nurse consultant Maureen Lagan; the Australian National

Health and Medical Research Council (NHMRC) for funding much of our research; and Allen & Unwin—in particular Elizabeth Weiss, Academic and Digital Publishing Director, for her steadfast encouragement and backing for this series of books, and copy editor Nicola Young, for a superb edit of the material.

Introduction

From blue to black and beyond

This book brings together the voices of women and their partners and family as they recount their experiences of pregnancy, birth and the first years with a young family. There are also observations from the other side of the desk provided by nurses, clinicians and counsellors. We have added our views, too. Just like this book, ideally, pregnancy and motherhood involve support and a team effort.

While most women find motherhood fulfilling, many also find the transition to becoming a mother more daunting than they had imagined. Most adjust well after a time; some continue to feel down or anxious. Depression and anxiety during the perinatal period are common and often transient, but more severe problems can go undetected or are not disclosed, and they have direct and indirect consequences. For that reason we look at how to recognise when a difficulty has become a disorder, and how to successfully manage the more distinctive mood disorders.

The key message of this book is that the perinatal disorders are very responsive to treatment and support.

We set the scene with stories from three eloquent women: one describing the baby blues, another the blackness of postnatal depression and the third a painful failure to bond with her baby—each account is worlds apart in causes, features and trajectories, but illustrating the differences between conditions that abate naturally with time and those that call for skilled management and support.

SHONA'S STORY: A BLUE VIEW

My preparation for the birth of my first child focused on the physical aspects. I anticipated pain. I expected hours of misery and yelling and hand clenching. I had predicted the way the birth should (or could) occur. It was to be a first child, so plenty of reading was done by me into the process. Of course, like any first mother-to-be I secretly hoped for a natural birth, leaving me exhilarated. But to others I admitted that I had no real birth plan; I conceded that no one can know how the birth would actually be.

But all of that preparation really was about the birth itself. Not so much of my knowledge related to afterwards. There was just a vague hope that my automatic mothering instincts would kick in.

Readers who have been in this situation can already perceive my naivety.

I am, in my professional career, a very able person. I completed my arts/law degree in record time whilst working almost full time as a law clerk and then stepped straight into the position of a country solicitor: a sink-or-swim world where I certainly swam. I had spent eight months devouring books on pregnancy, I went to all of the classes, and I asked questions of my treating doctor. I had googled every part of it.

Despite my research, an emergency caesarean was necessary; and despite my knowledge of the subject and my practicality in other realms of my existence, I was shattered that I had not been able to give birth myself. I am not sure I have yet forgiven myself, even though I know that it is nothing to be ashamed of.

Of course I had read about the baby blues and of postnatal depression. Everyone had taken the quiz at about 26 weeks. But in my life I had always been in control. I have a wonderful husband, a comfortable life, an understanding workplace. It made no sense to me that I would dip into such feelings. It was just irrational. Midwives had warned of the 'day 4 baby blues', a day when mothers suddenly start blubbering for no good reason, and I knew that it certainly would not happen to me.

From the time that I first really saw my baby, lying on my husband's hairy chest trying to suckle at out-of-action nipples, I truly loved her, though I also felt that there was already a part of her life (weighing her, the first cuddle) that I had missed out on because of the operation and recovery time. Despite this, breastfeeding came naturally, I started to come to terms with not having had a 'proper' birth, and I felt okay. Not the exhilaration that I had expected to feel, not that wonderful relief, but it was okay.

So I woke up on the fourth morning, still in hospital and sore from the caesarean, and immediately thought to myself, 'Well, I'm not depressed, I'm perfectly fine. I can now tick that box that says I have escaped the baby blues.'

Again, naive.

Since we had arrived at hospital (my husband stayed in the room with the baby and me), we had taken it in turns to order our hospital meals for the next day. The menu would arrive in the afternoon and we would tick meal options. The next morning, voilà, we would have meals that were almost similar to their description.

Well, the previous evening it had been my task to order the meals. I distinctly recall deliberating about which soup to pick, which snacks, and whether to go with roast beef or pork. What I do not distinctly recall doing was actually ticking those boxes.

Unfortunately, the only food that arrived at our door was one bowl of clear broth—to share for the entire day.

I dissolved into floods of tears. My husband laughed and said we'd order pizza, but to me it suddenly felt as if the entire world had broken down and nothing could possibly fix the huge mess that I had put our family in. And parallel to these feelings, I still also knew that it was silly to even be worried about it.

But there I was, unable to stop crying, crying so hard my shoulders were heaving. I thrust the baby at my husband and locked myself in the en suite. I sat on a chair and directed the water from the shower nozzle on me. And I couldn't stop crying. The mirror showed me my body in all its immediate devastation: a lumpy belly that still looked pregnant and a wound holding it together. It was truly a bizarre experience and I think I really worried my husband (standing, I am sure utterly confused, with the pizza menu in one hand and a hungry baby in the other, listening to his wife weeping in the bathroom).

I stayed in that bathroom, under that shower, for at least an hour. I only stopped when I thought I would be able to hold back my tears, but as soon as I started drying myself they started again. Deep breathing was no use, nor a warm face cloth. So I just sat for longer and each minute made it even more difficult for me to think of how to explain my behaviour.

Luckily, when I finally emerged from the bathroom, I was asked no questions. A simple, 'You okay?' (to which I burst into tears again) and then silence.

Now that was only the baby blues, and the next day my hormones must have become more stable. I was back to my old self. But that situation, where you have your mind telling you that this is ridiculous but your body is just absolutely freaking out, can happen to anybody.

I do not think that I recovered from the baby blues by anything more than mere luck. And luck is, of course, something that is not down to me. Had I spun that chocolate wheel another day, had a different genetic make-up, a 'difficult' baby, who knows what I may have felt or how long that state of mind may have lasted.

JULIETTE'S STORY: LOST AND FOUND

You stare at the damp stain on the ceiling through the grainy gloom of pre-dawn. You stare at the shape and trace it with your eyes and try to work out whether it is diminishing or getting larger. You realise that you've been staring at it wide-eyed every night since the baby came home. And that was the last time you slept—before the baby came home. Your husband is sleeping. Your 2-year-old and 4-year-old also. And yes, the baby is sleeping. There's a hush over the suburb. Even the cicadas are asleep, the night birds and the possums. It's possible you alone are the only person awake in the universe. And it's the same every night. Every night since you brought the baby home. Twelve weeks, but who's counting?

It's maybe 3 am or 4 or 5. Who would know? The world has slowed ever so slightly and time has lost its meaning. You are scratchy with fatigue and desperately want to sleep. But the stain is up there on the ceiling and you strain to make it out through the murky grey half-light. You hear the soft drumbeat of rain starting up, beating a gentle tattoo on the corrugated iron roof, and it sounds like tears to you. Someone is up there in the dark crying from the clouds. Someone besides you. You only cry at night when no one can see you, for what is there to cry about? Nothing. You have three bouncing children bursting with good health, a husband who is funny and works hard, a career you can go back to when ready, a house that's partly paid for, friends, family who love you, thoughtful neighbours, even a couple of goldfish to complete the domestic bliss.

But you hear the patter of the rain and you peer at the stain through the dancing shadows in the darkness to see if it's getting larger—and you think maybe it is. You can hear the rain coming down harder now and perhaps the roof is leaking and the water is seeping in through the tiles, trickling down the support beams, dripping into the insulation batts and soaking the plaster till it's sodden, till the whole ceiling is groaning with the weight of rainwater. And still it keeps raining, heavier now, and you wonder if the old Victorian ceiling is becoming like a giant sponge and might give way and fall on you, just sort of disintegrate, and huge chunks will fall from that great height and kill you in your bed. And you sort of welcome that thought, you sort of think that could be the answer, you wouldn't have to go through this anymore—this wretched sleepless emptiness, this wakeful nightmare that consumes you.

You think that if you were dead you could sleep and catch up on all those lost hours and it would be a sort of honourable death because it was an accident, a terrible accident. An old house, a faulty roof, an unstable ceiling. Who would have thought such a thing could happen? Let that be a lesson to us all. Go get your house checked, your roof, your beams, the electricals, everything ... And don't delay—who knows what type of time bomb you might be living with? And people would sniffle at the funeral and lament the loss of the gentle young mother and remember her with kind words and stirring hymns. They would rally to look after the three motherless children and the widowed young husband everybody loves, and bring around chicken casseroles and banana cakes, and take the two older ones to the park and wheel the baby around the block and offer to do the kindergarten run. And you know, they'd still be doing a better job than you. This is what you think in the dark hours before dawn.

The idea has appeal—a sort of sad haunting drama to it. A tender pathos. You listen to the tap, tap of the rain on the roof and you imagine the stain is growing before your bloodshot eyes and you consciously will the ceiling to fall in, to collapse upon you. You bid it to fall.

This is how it is.

Lost and found: you've lost the careless oblivion of motherhood, you've found an insidious doubt that corrodes your belief in your parenting. The black dog dips its paintbrush and daubs your life in blues and blacks and muted greys. You know you are pathetic and it's paralysing. It's like something has come loose from its moorings.

You take care to hide this; no one must know. Such shame. With the homecoming of the third child a steamroller has ploughed through your life, smashing your self-esteem, flattening your energy, mashing your confidence. And this terrible truth about you cannot be shared because it wasn't like this with the first two, the girls, when you shone radiant and were so super-efficient and ebullient with the great fortune of your much-blessed life. So how disloyal you are to this third child, the boy, who is such a good baby—everyone says so—to not enjoy him, to not remember when you last fed him (was it two hours or four?), to waver in indecision whether to bathe him or not because suddenly the task seems onerous and overwhelming, to feel so exhausted when he demands so little, and worse—to be so bereft of feeling for the little fellow?

And all of this makes you sad because you know you've been lucky in life and should be grateful, and you're not the sympathy-seeking type. You've always faced up to things, managed to snap yourself out of the doldrums. But this despair, this despondency, is like nothing you've ever known before. You realise it's here for good. This is your lot in life; you accept you will never be happy again. Not like you were, not so long ago. You weep at bandaid advertisements on television. You well up when a friend tells you her cat has died . . . and you hate cats, they give you asthma. You sob uncontrollably when a pedestrian abuses you because he thinks you've stopped too close to the crossing.

(You probably have: you're hopeless at driving now, like everything else.) You shed tears when a kindly soul offers you her place in the supermarket checkout queue.

You wonder if your baby will ever learn to talk because you're too tired to speak to him. The baby is thriving—everyone says so—but you feel as if he is sucking the life out of you. You are a robot, a mute automaton moving through the day, the hours dense and thickened like porridge, time erased. You've always put on a brave face, always managed—all the more reason you must struggle on alone now, lest someone suspects you're not coping. No one does. But if they did—then what? You are a mother with a mask but a lunatic gleam in her eye.

Then one day, you go to the doctor. For a papilloma on the sole of your foot that has been there for years. He's a friend of sorts, the doctor—your kids do swimming lessons together and you see him socially sometimes, at fundraising events for the kindy and the like. You don't really have a doctor because you don't get sick, but sometimes you need a referral to an obstetrician when you get pregnant, or to see someone when one of the kids has a fever.

He zaps the papilloma, but doesn't seem much interested in it. Instead, he looks at you intently for a long time and then says, 'You're not yourself, are you?'

Such a simple sentence. It's as if a light that's been switched off flickers on. Dim at first but soft and golden nonetheless. And so starts the long road back.

TAYLOR'S STORY: WHY WASN'T I TOLD?

My little new baby cried and cried and cried. I sat at the bottom of the garden facing the paling fence: the monster following grew larger with each wail. The old ladies of the neighbourhood asked what was wrong, their babies had never cried.

In my head, silent: 'She doesn't like me. I'm the wrong mother. Can I send her back?'

The clinic nurse checks her weight, suggests a little cereal, measures her and stamps her pink book.

'You need to play with her,' she says.

'Do I?'

My mind races. When might I do this? I'm not dressed until after lunch, then there's the mountain of small clothes and buckets of pooey nappies and when did I last eat? Her father will be home at some stage—though not early enough for me to walk around the block and down past the shops out past the point and into the ocean until I can't hear her anymore. He'll want something from me too and threaten to go elsewhere if he doesn't get it. And when is my trim figure returning?

I'm aged 24, armed with a degree in early childhood education: a baby should be a piece of cake—after all, they sleep most of the time. I'd read that in a book my mother gave me: 'Mother wakes at six o'clock. Nurse brings mother a cup of tea. Nurse brings baby to be fed. Mother bathes and has a good breakfast. Baby put in the fresh air for morning sleep. Mother naps after lunch. Nurse takes baby for an afternoon walk. Dinner is served at seven. Mother retires early for essential rest.'

When does help arrive?

It comes in the guise of her father's best friend, a bachelor longing for marriage and children of his own. She stops crying, looks at him and smiles. He tosses her in the air. Throws her higher and higher, maybe he'll miss as she falls. The eggshell skull with its tiny crater pulses under the wisp of hair.

'She's a beautiful baby,' he says. She crows and pleads for more.

A second bath soothes the witching hour. She flexes, floats, returns to the womb she remembers before she met me. She'd tried so hard to stay there, taking days to emerge and not before being dragged by the steel hands that pulled too hard.

'You can't pick her up for 24 hours. She can only be fed every four hours otherwise you'll make a rod for your own back.'

If I keep her mouth full she's quiet. The bowls of mush change from white to yellow to green, a bottle of fruit juice and then a start on cow's milk. Anyone can feed her now. She spits the breast as if I'm trying to poison her. The milk pours out, she's drowning.

Her dark eyes sum me up and find I'm lacking: 'You don't know what you're doing, do you?'

There's no money—one wage stretches only so far. Her father is *staying out later and later; he may never come home. Where did his beautiful girl go? Into a stained dressing gown that smells sour and covers too many cups of coffee, too much toast.*

The conversation stalls.

'Don't you want to know what she did today?'

'We're not ever going through this again,' he says. 'And by the way, I had to cancel the nappy service.'

I ask, 'I'd like you to hold her before you go to work so I can shower and dress. If I can get that done at least the day can begin.'

I make up a song for her: 'Girl, girl, pretty girl, from your head right to your toes.'

She considers it.

My baby and I walk for miles. Baby scowls at the sky, the trees and the faces. She's not sure but at least she's quiet.

The days begin to divide into meals, bathing and sleep. I must smile when I go to pick her up—she hasn't woken on purpose just to interrupt what I'm doing. She listens for the bachelor's footsteps, smiles saved like packets of rice packed away in her cheeks, the play so rough the little body quivers with delight as he tickles and tumbles. She's asleep when her father comes home.

'Could I go back to work early?' I plead with him.

'The sisters Kennedy mind babies up to 12 months old.' They're trained infant nurses. 'All meals cooked from scratch. Singing accompanied by the guitar,' says the brochure. We visit. Six babies sit contentedly in a circle, propped up in their chairs, the smell of baking, a soft breeze flutters the curtains. Everything is clean and starched.

Baby looks but reserves judgement.

Next week I drive into their street, dressed before nine, a new suit. We round the corner. She doesn't look at me, turns her head away. Their door opens, she stretches her arms out to be taken. I return at 3.30. Her head turns away.

'Mummy missed you. Did you have a lovely day?'

She sits on the floor and catches a bit of dust from the air. 'You'll have to work much harder than that,' she seems to say.

Imperceptibly, I come up for air. Now she can sit alone, hold a toy, sleep through the night, withstand the sight of her father—even with his glasses on. She's tumbling forward, rocking, she's on the move. She's cruising the furniture, helping arrange the books on the shelf and disappearing where no one will find her.

'Where's Blossom?'

'Here I are!'

My heart finally flips. I look into her eyes and fall in a rush. Am I too late? Will she forgive me?

What had gone so wrong? No one prepares you for the vacuum you'll be sucked into where you drown and lose everything you thought you were. You change your mind but there is no return. You've been a lover, a wife, a friend and a teacher—gone in a blink. Birth is a celebration the whole world knows how to do. They come with small, coloured gifts.

'Oh, she is so beautiful.'

Yes, but you can hardly believe it. For days you stare at her: it can't be possible that she belongs to you. But once home, how you long to be a well-wisher come for a brief visit. I think, 'I should never be left alone with her while you go back to your lives. It takes a village to raise a child.'

But I keep quiet.

* * *

And now I'm a grandmother: my chance to do better with her son— and I do. I visit each day. I tell her she's doing a good job. I clean and cook and send her to bed while I take him for a walk. I reassure her that it gets easier, breastfeeding takes weeks to establish, it's no time to think about dieting.

His daddy was at the birth, cut the cord and was the first to hold him. I thought I'd never get a go. He took weeks off work and kept the little body upright, close to his chest, soothing the grumbles away. He discovered a warm bath at any time of the day smoothed out the tiny furrowed face and the rigid belly.

She challenges the authority of the baby commandments. She begins to trust her own instincts and to stand her ground over co-sleeping, demand feeding and advice that doesn't ring true. This is her baby and she'll do it her way. He's gained weight, reached milestones—no harm has been done by not observing the 'rules'.

Visitors are welcome to see the baby, not the state of the house. The internet provides chat rooms where like-minded mothers can be found and ideas aired, the heaven and hell expressed in safety; if someone disapproves she can click them away.

'Why doesn't anyone tell you the truth?' she wails on a bad day.

And so we have an honest conversation about motherhood. I'd had many negative moments, so hers are allowed. Then we look at him sleeping and wonder how we could feel anything but overwhelming love. We laugh and I hug her tight.

Her saving is surrendering to what is happening and not trying to control too much.

One day at a time . . . until she wakes one morning: he's slept through the night . . . and then he smiles.

one

What are perinatal mood disorders?

*Advocates of industrial androgyny say pregnancy is not an illness.
Well, neither is busting a femur or ripping open a scrotum on a
fishhook, but that doesn't mean it's not a good idea to keep still for
a while afterwards.*

Emma Tom[1]

During pregnancy many women experience at least some depressive symptoms and around 10 per cent are at risk of developing a
clinical 'syndrome'. A similar number of women are affected during
the postnatal period, too. Following the birth, and particularly in the
next days or months, women are vulnerable to fluctuating moods,
including:
- the *baby blues*
- *depressive reactions* brought on by adjustment difficulties
- *non-melancholic depressive syndromes*, that is, as later depressions brought on by the stressful situation rather than caused
  by a chemical imbalance in the body

and several more biological conditions (that is, those caused by
chemical imbalances rather than stress, although they can still be be
worsened by stress), including:
- *melancholia* or *melancholic depression*
- *puerperal psychosis* (or *psychotic depression*)
- *bipolar disorder.*

Postnatal depression (PND) is usually non-melancholic (that is, caused by stress rather than a chemical imbalance) but in about 10 per cent of cases is melancholic (for more, see 'Postnatal depression' below). Postnatal disorders can, while present and if severe, interfere with the bonding and attachment of mother and her baby and impose strains upon the parents' relationship, as well as cause distress to the new mother herself. A depressive episode is also marked by decreased confidence, which can create secondary problems, and may also drive feelings of irritability and anger. All such mood disorders—apart from the baby blues and puerperal psychosis—can occur at other times of life and display the same clinical features, but doctors will tailor their treatment choices differently when a woman is pregnant or breastfeeding.

The following 'map' of the perinatal mood disorders may help you determine whether you're in the territory of perinatal mood disorders or not. The geography of motherland seems deceptively familiar until you get there.

THE TERM 'PERINATAL'

In this book we use the term *perinatal* to refer to the time from the start of pregnancy to the end of the baby's first year.

The strict definition used for statistical purposes by the Australian Institute of Health and Welfare[2] classifies the perinatal period as starting at 20 completed weeks of gestation and ending at 28 completed days after birth.

DEPRESSION: AN OVERVIEW

One day I was at home alone with the kids. I was exhausted and on the verge of tears. My 3-year-old climbed onto my lap and took my face in his chubby little hands and said, 'Don't worry, Mummy.' It was my awakening. At last I could admit to myself that I had a problem.

Zara

'Depression' is a word that is used loosely. It is used to describe everything from mood states to economic recessions, so a diagnosis of depression is diffuse and liable to variable interpretation and misinterpretation. Depression is, in essence, a term more comparable with 'pain'. It is a marker of superficially similar but actually quite diverse entities. When the term 'depression' is used to describe a mood state it needs to be more closely defined. For instance, it is important to differentiate between 'normal' depression (or everyday temporary unhappiness) and clinical depression—in the same way a dermatologist would be expected to distinguish a benign mole from a melanoma—as it influences the type and success of treatment.

Signs and symptoms of depression

Someone with depression feels down and hopeless, helpless and pessimistic, but one key symptom is a drop in self-esteem and, correlated with that, an increase in self-criticism. This decline in self-regard distinguishes depression from other conditions such as grief, sadness or anxiety.

Grief is the distress felt following usually irretrievable loss and separation, when an attachment bond is broken. While grief can be severe and disabling, it is not accompanied by a drop in self-esteem. *Sadness* is an emotional reaction to losses or disappointments, a feeling of being down and unhappy, that dissipates within days and self-worth is rarely diminished. *Anxiety* is essentially a state of insecurity or fear and hyper-arousal. People with depression (including PND) are frequently anxious (and anxiety can set the stage for depression), and some people who are grieving will later develop depression, but clarifying the primary emotional state is the best way towards effective treatment.

The Edinburgh postnatal depression scale (EPDS; see Chapter 3) is a widely used screening instrument for postnatal depression. As the instrument includes anxiety as well as depression items, a percentage who score positive will do so due to having a primary anxiety rather than a primary depressive condition during the postnatal period.

ANXIETY AND PANIC ATTACKS

A new mother has to traverse some very unfamiliar territory, which can be more than somewhat overwhelming. Many women already have lifelong anxious tendencies, but when anxiety becomes more prevalent than feelings of wellbeing, something else is going on. As many of our essayists attest, a baby provides a focus for intense worry and anxiety-based preoccupations.

Most people never experience a *panic attack*, although they would recognise the symptoms, which are the feelings people experience when they're frightened or under threat—the so-called 'flight or fight' response. A panic attack seems to come from nowhere, though. Feelings of panic and terror build up and intensify to such a degree that the sufferer may feel like they're having a heart attack or a stroke or like they're literally going to die. Symptoms include tightness in the chest, chest pains, a racing heart, dizziness and breathing too fast, tingling all over, numbness, weakness, sweating and muscle cramps. A panic attack is so unpleasant that it can create a feedback loop, where feelings of panic increase the feelings of panic. Nevertheless, people can have panic attacks and not recognise them as being a symptom of a mood disorder. They think they're going mad or have some terrible physical disorder but don't consider the attack as indicating that something is *psychologically* wrong, since panic attacks are so awfully physical. Poorly understood or untreated panic can result in secondary symptoms, particularly depression and phobic avoidance. Avoidance responses often take the form of a disabling mantra, such as, 'What if [*insert disastrous event*] occurs?', which can lead to fear of even leaving the house.

In addition to panic attacks, women who have an anxious, worrying temperament can experience increased anxiety during the postnatal period, and *obsessive-compulsive disorder* (OCD) can worsen—or emerge for the first time.

Such anxiety states generally benefit from different treatment from those used to manage the depressive conditions. This is another good reason to seek out a competent clinical assessment to identify your primary condition.

'Normal' depression

Depression can, in fact, be normal. Experiencing a depressed mood (that is, feeling down, experiencing lowered self-esteem, feeling like giving up) is a universal human experience, but such states are generally brief, lasting from hours to days, lift of their own accord or respond to pleasant events, and do not disrupt normal living. While there is no distinct boundary between a depressed mood and clinical depression, the latter is more severe and persistent, unlikely to lift by itself and associated with distinctive features. Clinical depressive conditions are highly likely to benefit from tailored professional assistance.

STRESSORS

A stressor is an event or interpersonal interaction that causes distress. Stressors can be acute (that is, short-term, such as the immediate aftermath of an accident) or chronic (that is, ongoing, such as poverty or a poor marriage). They cause strain that can distort personality development and lead to anxiety and depression. Psychologists define stressors in the sufferer's recent and/or current life as *proximal stressors* and those in the sufferer's past as *distal stressors*.

For more on stressors, see Chapter 2.

Clinical depression

Non-melancholic depressive disorders

The *non-melancholic depressive disorders* are made up of a raft of depressive disorders arising from the impact of personally relevant stressors on individual personality styles, and lack specific defining features. While people suffering from non-melancholic depression may be severely (even suicidally) depressed, there is usually some reactivity in their mood (that is, they can be cheered up in certain circumstances) and they can experience some level of pleasure in life (even if reduced). Psychomotor disturbance (see box below), a key feature of melancholia, is absent. Sleep disturbance is more likely to involve difficulty in getting to sleep or patchy sleep (and even excessive sleeping) rather than early morning wakening.

PSYCHOMOTOR DISTURBANCE

'Psychomotor' is a word used in medicine to describe the link between mental processes and physical movements. In depression, neural connections can become disturbed, leading either to 'retardation' or 'agitation'. Retardation is characterised by slowed thinking, walking and speech, a lack of energy for even the most basic tasks (called anergia) and poor concentration and memory. Agitation is characterised by excessive worrying and morbid ruminations, and physical symptoms such as pacing the floor, a churning stomach and racing thoughts that may be perplexed and full of foreboding (such as 'What will become of me?').

In comparison to melancholia, a depression underpinned by biological changes such as imbalances in brain chemicals, the clinical patterns of non-melancholic depression are determined by its causes and are relatively non-specific. For example, a woman with an anxious, worrying temperament may, when depressed, internalise her anxiety by worrying more and isolating herself from others, or externalise her anxiety via irritability and anger.

The majority of perinatal depressive disorders are non-melancholic. Pregnancy and the postnatal interval provide many potential stressors that can lead to non-melancholic depressions such as adjustment disorder, and situational and reactive depressions. These tend to resolve over time as the sufferer adapts to the stressors, unless there are maintaining factors in their life. That is not to say, however, that we would ever advise simply waiting for a depressive disorder to lift naturally. Left untreated, such a depression can cause impairment that at this crucial time is likely to have significant influence both on the mother's mental and physical health and on the psychological wellbeing of her whole family.

Non-melancholic depressions respond well to psychological strategies, although medication is of benefit when symptoms are severe, or to address some symptoms (such as restoring sleep or muting anxiety). For more on the principal types of non-melancholic depression—and differing management suggestions—see the Black Dog website[3] and our book by Gordon Parker and Vijaya Manicavasagar, *Modelling and Managing the Depressive Disorders: A Clinical Guide.*[4]

Melancholic depression

Medical intervention is needed to treat melancholic depression or melancholia (once known as endogenous depression). This type of depression is more distinctly biological (that is, caused by changes in brain chemistry rather than external stressors), is unlikely to lift on its own and may take a long time to improve without medical treatment. Postnatal melancholia has a distinct pattern of symptoms (see below) and generally appears within four weeks of the birth. Riley's story illustrates a common pattern:

> *I ended up having an emergency caesarean. When I got to hold my baby I was completely underwhelmed. I remember the nurses kept having to put the baby back on my chest as I was kind of holding her like a football under one arm and she was slipping off the bed. When my own mother called all I could say was that the baby had hairy shoulders. Intellectually, I could see that she was stunningly beautiful and physically perfect, but emotionally, it just wasn't registering.*
>
> *People told me a lot of my feelings were probably due to the caesar, so I gave myself time to recover but it never got brighter. My whole life was stained with grey . . . like limp wet washing with no sun or breeze. I was slowed down, listless, no appetite, awake from the crack of dawn though so exhausted. I struggled with everything. Not just with the baby but absolutely everything: news bulletins, road signs, phone conversations. It was like coming out of hospital and everyone was speaking Japanese. My whole world had literally changed. I had changed. And while I coped with that I was supposed to look after a baby as well? Motherhood was monotonous and joyless and terrifying. But when I tried to explain what was happening it just came across as so silly, though by this stage even my voice sounded peculiar to me.*

The principal clinical feature of melancholic depression is psycho-motor disturbance. The chance of a melancholic PND is increased in women who have had episodes of melancholic depression in the past or who have a family history of melancholia.

Features of melancholic depression include:

- over-represented symptoms and signs (that is, more prominent than you would expect for depression in general) (see below)
- a family history of melancholic depression (that is, a genetic predisposition)
- changes in sleep patterns, circadian rhythms (that is, bodily responses to the time of day) and brain neurotransmitters (messenger molecules)
- a better response to physical treatments (that is, antidepressant medication) than to psychotherapy or counselling.

Management of melancholic depression (see Chapter 10) generally involves medication initially, and then a set of non-medication strategies (such as psychotherapy or counselling) to address illness-related problems or to maintain recovery.

Symptoms of melancholic depression include:

- psychomotor disturbance—see box above.
- an 'anhedonic' and non-reactive mood—a lack of pleasure (called anhedonia) in present or anticipated activities, and no lift in mood in response to positive events. Such symptoms may be either absolute (unchanging) or partial ('I guess seeing my child lifts my mood somewhat'), and either continuous or relieved only briefly ('Seeing my child gives me some pleasure but it doesn't last').
- diurnal variation of mood and energy—changes in energy and mood in response to the time of day or night, in particular being worse in the morning.
- non-specific features—including early morning waking, and loss of weight and appetite.

Although melancholic depression was once thought to emerge without any obvious precipitant or in response to only a minor trigger, we now recognise that stress may bring on melancholic depression—particularly the first episode. The depressive response is, however, generally more severe, persistent and out of proportion to the stressor.

Melancholic depression is slightly more likely in women with an obsessional or stoic personality style, who then commonly conceal their symptoms. Actor Brooke Shields provides a poignant account in her book *Down Came the Rain*.[5]

Psychotic depression

Psychotic depression has a melancholia base. Its key features are psychomotor disturbance and an anhedonic and non-reactive mood (described above). However, diurnal variation in mood and energy (that is, across the day) are not necessarily present with both compromised across the day. Psychomotor disturbance is usually more severe than in melancholia, and observable to others. Someone with psychomotor retardation may just lie in bed or slump in a chair and have minimal interaction with others—while many develop constipation as their bodily processes slow down. In addition, sufferers have psychotic experiences, losing touch with reality through delusions (false beliefs) and/or hallucinations (seeing or hearing things that aren't there, or experiencing abnormally heightened senses of taste and smell).

In a postnatal psychotic state the mother may feel that she and her baby have no future and would be better off dead. While psychotic depression is uncommon, if it occurs postnatally it is often described as a *puerperal psychosis* and is treated as a psychiatric emergency.

PERINATAL DEPRESSION AND ANXIETY: AN OVERVIEW

The baby blues

Up to 80 per cent of new mothers develop the baby blues as their hormones fluctuate and oestrogen and progesterone levels drop sharply after birth. The baby blues generally come on three to six days after birth (though earlier if the birth has been difficult), and while some episodes end naturally in a matter of hours, most do so by around two weeks after birth. They are slightly more likely to be experienced by second-time mothers than those having their first baby.[6]

Though the baby blues are distressing and associated with many depressive symptoms, they do not constitute a psychiatric disorder. They are also widely experienced and transient.

The most common symptoms include:

- being overly emotional and changeable in spirits (having what doctors call a labile mood)
- crying (often unable to stop) or feeling tearful
- being oversensitive
- tiredness and fatigue
- inability to concentrate—getting forgetful and muddled
- irritability, anxiety and feeling tense
- sadness, low spirits and a depressed mood
- inability to show feelings
- insomnia, despite feeling exhausted.

During such episodes many women also report intervals of happiness, calmness, liveliness and confidence, so that the baby blues are better viewed as changeable, unsteady and easily altered emotions rather than a constant down mood. In essence, they are a state of emotional dysregulation that dissipates within a few days.

Postnatal depression (PND)

Postnatal depression (PND) is a generic diagnostic term applied to many postnatal conditions but does not include the baby blues. PND encompasses the more severe, disabling and/or prolonged states of clinical depression that interfere with the ability to function (for example, hampering the mother's capacity to look after the baby). The term is sometimes applied to describe women for whom the primary problem is anxiety, rather than depression per se, since some of the assessment tools used to aid diagnosis include many symptoms of anxiety. Is it anxiety or depression or a mixture? (See earlier in this chapter for the difference between anxiety and depression.) The answer depends on the individual case and requires assessment by a competent health professional. Depression and anxiety both benefit from tailored treatment approaches which respect disorder-specific differences as well as commonalities.

Studies examining the rates of PND in the community estimate the general risk of developing PND as 10–20 per cent. A classic review of the scientific literature[7] quantified PND at 13 per cent, indicating that as many as one in eight women experience an episode after birth. Several factors increase the risk of PND: lower social status, more life stressors during pregnancy (see Chapter 2), a more difficult than normal pregnancy or delivery, relationship difficulties, lack of social support and previous episodes of depression and anxiety.

The period of greatest risk for melancholic depression (about 10 per cent of PND cases) is during the first four weeks after the birth. Episodes of non-melancholic depression come on more gradually, in the first three months, but a depressive disorder can develop any time up to a year after the baby's birth. If untreated, such episodes tend to last months or years.

Fathers are not immune to stress in the transition to fatherhood, either. Studies indicate high rates of psychological distress in around one in five expectant fathers. Issues of adjustment to the new role and lifestyle make a distinct contribution, and stress is also associated with a poor marital relationship and poor social networks. As well, fathers who have insufficient information about pregnancy and childbirth are at greater risk of distress. Such realities highlight the obvious need to include fathers in the processes of pregnancy and birth and to ensure that they remain informed about their partner's pregnancy and childbirth and issues to do with caring for a newborn.[8] For more on fathers and perinatal mood conditions, see Chapter 11.

Puerperal psychosis

I had lost 10 kilograms in the six weeks since leaving hospital with our baby. I was still on a high; in fact I believed that I could write lots of books what with all these fantastic ideas flooding my thoughts. The next week I remember one night when I just sat and watched my little daughter sleeping, waiting for her to wake for a feed. She slept all through the night while I just sat there with my thoughts keeping me occupied until sunrise.

I was no longer sleeping or eating and I could hear people speaking to me, only they weren't there. To me it was like there was a reel of film playing in my head and it played my thoughts over and over from one extreme to the other: from ecstasy to grief and devastation then back to ecstasy in the same minute, over and over and over.

I recall the day I was hospitalised. It was a very hot day, I had bare feet, the reel of film playing in my head, and I was apparently walking in the middle of a busy highway while swinging my naked baby around in the air. The voices I was hearing were telling me that the world was ending but that it was okay because we were all going together and nothing would hurt anymore. I remember a car screeching near my feet. After several unsuccessful attempts by people pulling over and trying to help, I was apprehended by police and taken to hospital.

I found out later that my daughter was taken to hospital by ambulance and treated for dehydration and sunburn. There is no way for me to describe how this event makes me feel. I nearly ended my daughter's little life.

Sophia

Puerperal psychosis, also known as postpartum psychosis, is a condition characterised by psychotic symptoms (hearing 'voices' or having delusional ideas), along with symptoms of severe depression or mania or a mixture of the two. Postnatal psychotic depression is a form of puerperal psychosis (see above). In this condition, the psychotic symptoms are more overtly bizarre and disturbing. Puerperal psychosis usually comes on rapidly—often in the first 48 hours after childbirth—but can occur any time in the first month. The overall risk is low (1–2 women in every 1000 deliveries, or 0.1–0.2 per cent).

It is more likely to occur in women who have a family history of melancholic or psychotic depression or bipolar disorder and/or who have experienced such episodes in the past.[9] People experiencing such states are variably diagnosed as having stress-induced psychosis (called psychogenic psychosis), psychotic depression, mania, schizophrenia or mixed states. Follow-up studies show, however, that most have a bipolar disorder (see below). Sophia, in the story above, for instance, said that she was 'still on a high' after being discharged from hospital. In such cases, the bipolar disorder is triggered by childbirth. It is almost unheard of for women experiencing a puerperal psychosis to go on to develop schizophrenia.[10]

Symptoms of puerperal psychosis include the following:

- severe insomnia
- confusion or perplexity
- fearfulness
- delusions of grandeur
- guilt
- paranoia
- worthlessness
- preoccupations that the baby is ill or dying
- psychomotor disturbance—retardation or agitation
- distrust of other people.

A characteristic feature of puerperal psychosis is confusion or perplexity, with each also being key features of delirium (a brain syndrome that develops when brain function is compromised, such as when an individual has a fever). This led to speculation that puerperal psychosis was linked to puerperal fever (the result of infection) but this is not the case. What it does suggest is that there is some brain dysfunction, triggered by childbirth, linked to puerperal psychosis and that some aspects are a response to changes in the body after the birth. It could reflect a shift in the hypothalamic–pituitary–adrenal (HPA) axis which, via feedback from body systems, controls hormonal and nervous system activity and regulates mood and emotion and changes in other biological systems.

As a consequence of such a florid (fully present) psychotic condition, the woman is at high risk of harm and, at times, her baby can also be at risk. Puerperal psychosis carries a 5 per cent suicide rate and a 4 per cent infanticide rate, and is seen as a psychiatric emergency. It generally involves hospitalisation and treatment with antipsychotic medication. Electroconvulsive therapy (ECT) may also rapidly resolve the illness but is generally reserved for those who have not responded to medication or because of the severity of the state and the risk to the mother.

Bipolar disorder

My pregnancy was great; all my family and friends said I glowed with health. I was so happy to be pregnant. I was unaware of any underlying mental illness. Towards the end I started to become quite tired but could not sleep, but I dismissed this as a symptom of pregnancy. I delivered a healthy boy and though completely drained after many hours of labour I still didn't sleep—I couldn't. After a few days of sleeplessness I became confused about how to look after my newborn; it was at this point I knew something was wrong. The nurses were concerned and referred me for psychological assessment. I was then sent to the local psychiatric hospital. The first day there I felt like a wild animal running from place to place. I had no idea where I was, or why I was there. Unsurprisingly, I still did not sleep.

The next day a psychiatrist evaluated me. She was a very kind and compassionate woman. She recommended that I be transferred from the locked ward to the mother-and-baby unit. There was a psychiatric nurse for me and a mothercraft nurse for my son. It was the weekend but they transferred me that morning. Nothing can describe the happiness I felt when I realised I hadn't hurt my son—I was so disoriented that I thought I might have harmed him.

The doctors diagnosed me with bipolar I disorder. People with this condition are more likely to experience mania for long periods of time and display psychotic symptoms. Months later my behaviour was described to me: I would start to do something like make a coffee then stop midway through to switch tasks, for example have a shower, and I continued to do this every five minutes throughout the day and some of the night.

After weeks of treatment I started to come out of the haze of manic psychosis into being, as the psychiatrist stated, 'only slightly unwell'. I was still misty with hypomania and I was writing a lot in my diary and on scraps of paper, and trying to grab hold of what day it was. I was still confused as to what was happening to me and why. I was slow to bond with my son but I gradually came to the realisation that I was a good mother who happened to have a mental illness. The staff also helped me understand that medication was the only way to help control the irrational thoughts I was having.

Sienna

The bipolar disorders are divided into two main subtypes—*bipolar I* and *bipolar II*. In bipolar I disorder—previously known as manic depression—the sufferer experiences psychotic manic episodes usually involving grandiose delusions and/or hallucinations (which are occasionally paranoid in content). These manic highs alternate with depressive episodes (most likely psychotic or melancholic depression).

Bipolar II disorder is the diagnosis reserved for those bipolar patients who never experience psychotic highs or lows, yet still have mood and energy swings, moving through hypomania (a less extreme high, and without psychotic features) to melancholic depressive episodes. Some experience mixed states—a psychologically painful overlap of mania and depression, or rapid cycling—where their mood rapidly oscillates from the hypomanic pole to the depressed pole.

During screening at the Black Dog Institute, people who have experienced clinical depression are asked whether there are times, when they're not depressed, that they feel distinctly wired and ener-gised. If they answer yes, then we investigate other features of their highs in order to move towards a correct diagnosis.

The following features suggest a diagnosis of bipolar disorder:

- being over-talkative, garrulous, loud
- overspending, especially buying things that can't be afforded
- sleeping less but not feeling tired
- feeling more creative, special, talented, entitled
- feeling indestructible, bulletproof
- having increased libido
- a dissipation of anxiety, feeling carefree and playful
- indiscretion, lack of caution, with no filtering of what is said or done.

Subtyping into bipolar type I or II depends on whether or not the highs have psychotic features. There is often a clear point (called a trend break) of bipolar onset—a time when such episodes emerged for the first time and were a distinct change from normal functioning. For those with a bipolar II disorder, this commonly occurs during adolescence, while it is somewhat later for those with a bipolar I condition. A high percentage of people with a bipolar disorder will have a family member with a history of bipolar or clinical depression, which implies a strong genetic component.

Women with bipolar disorder are at a 50–60 per cent increased risk of developing a postnatal mood state, be it a high or a depression. Women with a family history of bipolar disorder who have never personally experienced bipolar mood swings are at increased risk of a first episode after the birth.

Postnatal hypomania tends to occur in the first day or two following birth (compared to days 3–5 for the baby blues) but should not be diagnosed simply on the basis of mood symptoms such as elation (some level of euphoria is felt by most women after having a baby). Accurate diagnosis requires reference to the symptoms listed above and that such symptoms be distinctive, even if not severe.

For women who have been taking antidepressant medication during pregnancy hypomanic symptoms can be induced by their medication. In such cases they are diagnosed as having a 'bipolar III' state, which means they don't necessarily have a bipolar II condition, but symptoms that look like bipolar disorder have been induced by the introduction or increased dose of the antidepressant medication.

Bipolar disorder in the perinatal period carries special challenges, especially with regard to the use and safety of preventative (termed prophylactic) mood stabilisers during pregnancy and if the mother wishes to breastfeed. It is essential that a correct diagnosis is made in such cases, so that appropriate treatment strategies can be developed and women are not needlessly put on medication if their condition is not, in fact, a bipolar disorder. See the Appendix for more detail on medication types, effectiveness and safety.

MORE INFORMATION

The Black Dog Institute's website has an overview of bipolar conditions,[11] our book *Bipolar II Disorder: Modelling, Measuring and Managing* gives a detailed overview of bipolar II disorder and its management[12] and our website has a self-test for depression both during pregnancy and after the birth—as well as a self-test for bipolar disorder.[13] All the self-tests on our website can be completed anonymously.

Accurate detection and diagnosis of mood disorder types (or at least a good working hypothesis to start from) is essential so that treatment can be matched to causes and ensure the best possible success. Later chapters provide further details about reaching a diagnosis, formulating a management plan and following a care pathway.

TEN KEY MESSAGES TO TAKE AWAY

This is the birthplace of hope. If you develop a mood disorder during the perinatal period you should confidently expect that it will be brought under control with appropriate assistance. And, equally importantly, in the process you will learn something about yourself and become more finely forged, resilient and wise in the face of life's stressors. Bear these points in mind as you read this book and as you take your motherhood journey.

1   Find out about perinatal depression and its various signs and symptoms.

2   Don't assume that you won't get perinatal depression—you can and may. Have someone else on watch too—the nature of a mood disorder is that you may not recognise it yourself.

3   If you find yourself struggling after the birth, admit it and seek help—and do so immediately.

4   Understand that you are in no way to blame for your mood disorder so don't allow yourself to feel any guilt. It is not only for yourself that you need to find help quickly—it is for your baby and your family as well.

5   Reject any feelings of stigma about developing a mood disorder at this time. It is much more common than most imagine.

6   Get the best professional help available to get you back to health. Seek a clear diagnosis and a management plan for working as a team.

7   Ask for help from your family and friends. They want to contribute.

8   Never doubt that you will fully recover.

9   Know that your baby and its bond with you will not be affected if you seek treatment for your mood disorder.

10 If you wish to have another child, know that you will not necessarily have perinatal depression again, but try to understand the causes of the episode you did have and what professional and family supports benefited your recovery. Have those supports in place for your next pregnancy anyway, just in case.

two

Risk factors for perinatal mood problems

My mum came to look after Zac while I went to the post office. I then walked across to the beach and opened the mail, whereupon a gust of wind blew his birth certificate out of my hand and I ended up chasing it across the beach, sobbing and wailing like a banshee.

Natalie

In this chapter we provide an overview of risk factors that can increase a woman's vulnerability to a mood disorder during pregnancy and, in particular, after the birth. We want to make clear at this point that while a risk factor indicates vulnerability, it *doesn't* necessarily mean that person will develop the specific condition.[1] In fact, knowledge also provides opportunity. If women are aware of their personal risk factors, they can adopt strategies to lower that risk.

Consider the following letter received from an acquaintance by a GP. Max emailed the GP when he realised that his wife, Jose, had become distressed past the point where she could stay on top of things using her usual ways of coping. He also understood that he was too close to the problem, indeed that he might be part of it, and that they both needed the steady hand of a professional who had seen it all before and would understand how to alleviate the mounting distress in the family.

Dear _____

Please excuse my contacting you but a difficult situation has arisen and I am at a loss about who to turn to.

It is about my wife. As you know, Jose and I have been married for eight years and have a daughter (Estrellita, 4) and now the new baby, Alejandro, born ten weeks ago. Estrellita is healthy and the baby eats and sleeps well.

I need to fill in some background for you . . .

Jose has just turned 35 (to my 57!). We met in Manila when I was working at the Asian Development Bank. She was (is) beautiful, of course, but was also a fiercely competent PA to my immediate superior at the bank. His 'right arm', he called her. She is the stand-out in her family. She is the eldest, then come four boys (a fifth died) and another girl. While two of her brothers are teachers and one a chauffeur, the remaining brother is a hopeless alcoholic and was diagnosed years ago as having a bipolar disorder (refused treatment). Jose has always been the family's rock. Her mother was widowed early and Jose has been the main breadwinner and scholarship-winner. The family came from a poor area of Manila and twice lost everything to floods, which also drowned her youngest brother when Jose was 6 years old. They are devout Catholics but she only observes when she is home visiting them. They are tough, dignified, and very hardworking and family-minded. You can imagine what a wrench it was for Jose to come back with me to Australia when we married. She goes back home to Manila at Easter each year and has taken Estrellita there twice.

Jose's mother had a serious fall in August and has had to give up her cleaning job. The concussion seems to have caused continuing giddiness and headaches and she now lives with her oldest son. Jose has been very worried about her. They have a complex relationship and seem to clash a lot, but they are close nonetheless. As you can imagine, this was not the best lead-in to the last few months of Jose's pregnancy. She has felt very torn but as she and I have discussed, there is nothing she can do to help her mother further at present. We have ensured that she has had the best medical treatment and we also provide significant financial support.

I have noticed over the years of our marriage that Jose has had what I'd call significant sadness from time to time, but her background and culture give little time or opportunity to examine such feelings. Her solution is to throw herself with quite ferocious energy into the endless tasks of raising a family. She is a loving though somewhat reserved mother. She keeps the home impeccable and is very house proud.

After the joys of our courtship, she has become private, task-focused and what I'd call emotionally cautious. She is dutiful and warm but occasionally I can sense that her heart is not in it. It's almost as if she's wearing a mask and is on autopilot, imitating what a person who is in her position would be doing. It has been a long time, now that I think of it, that I've seen her actually laugh.

I have been aware that she is becoming sadder, probably even depressed. She seems to have trouble getting the energy to keep up with a busy household and over the last year she has grown quieter. She has been going to the doctor for back and neck pain recently and visits an alternative medicine group for various herbs. Certainly she has not wanted to talk about any difficulties, just saying that two children would make anyone tired and that she's fine. She has been rather short with our daughter recently and once, when I came home from work early, I found Estrellita in tears, which was distressing.

In the last weeks, though, I have felt that Jose is really struggling. I have found her in tears twice and she has been spending more time in bed. One particularly worrying thing happened last Wednesday morning. At about 3 am as I got up to go to the bathroom, I noticed that she was wide awake and just lying there. When I asked if she was all right she said something that sounded like, 'I don't think I can do this anymore.' I couldn't be sure what she'd said and I was shocked, so asked her to repeat it. She just said that she was being silly and she'd be okay after some sleep but that she couldn't fall asleep again after Alejandro's feed though she was very tired.

Since Wednesday she has improved a bit, at least on the surface, but I think she's putting on a brave face. I know she needs help. There are enough clues. I think she won't resist help now if it's put in the right way. That sounds picky, but I know how sensitive she is and how she prides herself on being 'together'. The idea of being told she's got depression and needs treatment will put her right on the defensive and she'll likely fake good health. She, I think, will resist the idea that she might have a mental illness—people who have depression should just 'pull themselves together'. That's why I think it's time to visit a specialist who's seen it all before and can talk about it in the right way. Sadly, I think I'm part of her problem and I am certainly too close to it all.

So, in summary, I am really worried about Jose and would appreciate any advice you might have.

Max

WHAT'S GOING ON?

Different readers of this story are likely to focus on one particular risk factor or stressor and judge it to be central to Jose's distress. Some may suggest that being a new mother has taken away her senior work identity while others might nominate problems with her mother. Diagnostically, some might say the issue is an adjustment reaction to differing stressors while others might suspect a melancholic condition in light of her symptoms and the fact that one of her brothers possibly has bipolar disorder.

Treatment decisions are all contingent on identifying the most likely diagnosis and key contributors, and could lead to quite differing outcomes—medication, counselling or psychotherapy—and therapists (for example, GP, psychologist, psychiatrist or counsellor). Sophisticated professional assessment is vital in this and all cases to identify diagnostic issues, the most likely causes and the most considered approach to management. We will return to Jose's story in Chapter 4.

Jose's vignette is an introduction to the *biopsychosocial model* (outlined below) that can be applied to the postnatal disorders and to the many risk factors that can initiate and/or prolong them.

THE BIOPSYCHOSOCIAL MODEL FOR PERINATAL MOOD DISORDER RISK FACTORS

If it's five o'clock and the children are still alive—I've done my job.

Roseanne

Risk factors can broadly be grouped under the headings biological, psychological and social. They may play a role singly or in combination. If a combination (most commonly), the diagnostician's task is to identify the primary factor so that treatment and management strategies can be tailored to it.

Biological risk factors

Insanity is hereditary—you can get it from your children.

Sam Levinson

The biological risk factors for perinatal depression are very broad and all can lower the threshold for developing a mood disorder. We note only some of them here, with relevant examples. They include:

- a family or personal history of psychiatric or physical disorders (that is, a genetic predisposition)
- debilitating physical symptoms during pregnancy (such as severe nausea and vomiting)
- lack of physical fitness or poor general health (for example, anaemia, dietary imbalance)
- hormonal influences (especially a thyroid imbalance—PND doesn't necessarily arise from hormonal changes related to childbirth; a small proportion of women—those who are more prone to premenstrual syndrome [PMS]—seem to be at increased risk, perhaps due to oestrogen sensitivity)
- medications, especially psychotropic (mood-altering) medication, but also long-acting hormone-based contraceptives, as well as certain illicit drugs and high alcohol use
- a caesarean section (and the anaesthetic used) or a traumatic delivery
- extreme fatigue or insomnia during the postnatal period.

A pre-existing mood disorder

Already having a mood disorder (especially a bipolar condition), or a family history of mood disorders, is a potent risk factor for postnatal depression (PND) or for an elevated (for example, manic or hypo-manic) mood state.

Maria provides an example. She had suffered from depression and anxiety since she was 16 and had always been proactive in seeking treatment and help. She'd had a lot to deal with over the years, including struggles with alcohol, a divorce and then years of infertility. When, at 35 and happily remarried, she found she was pregnant, she was delighted. Finally she would become a mother after eight years of trying. She wrote:

Everyone knows about postnatal depression, but what happens if you already have depression? Do you get a double dose? I was on anti-depressants before I got pregnant and was advised not to stop them. I was assured the risks to the baby would be minimal and that not taking them would probably be more harmful for us both.

I was very concerned about how I would be after the birth and feared not being able to cope. I brought up my concerns with my GP, who sent a referral to the antenatal clinic. They organised an appoint-ment with a counsellor, where I discussed all my concerns and fears. She suggested I get assistance after the birth via regular home visits from a health nurse.

My husband was very supportive but as neither of us has family around we felt isolated and lonely. I found the visits from the nurse very helpful in alleviating my anxiety, as she visited weekly for about three months, then fortnightly and then monthly, until Toby was 12 months old. Any concern I had, especially in those first few weeks, I would write down and bring up at each visit, which stopped me from panicking and rushing to the doctors every time I was worried.

I also used the 13HEALTH[2] phone service regularly, especially during the pregnancy. I tend to worry far too much, which then worsens the depression and anxiety, so I found these services very useful and would definitely recommend them to other depression sufferers.

My depression did get worse after the birth, but having services already in place really did help. The nurse was then able to organise extra help—as I was struggling, especially in those first few months. There were also fortnightly home visits from a counsellor. I found it very hard to get out of the house early on and so the home visiting was much appreciated. There was also a family service volunteer who would visit weekly and we would go for a walk or meet for a coffee and discuss other things I could do.

It took about 12 months to really get used to my new role as a mum and to feel somewhat confident. That was about the time we started attending playgroups and meeting new people. But without outside help I would not have got through it as well as I did.

As noted earlier, having a pre-existing mental illness (especially a bipolar disorder) increases the chance of developing a perinatal mood disorder during pregnancy or after the birth. In such cases, it is important to make decisions about what psychotropic (mood-altering) medications to take during pregnancy to lower such risks. The mother and her partner, in discussion with an informed physician—psychiatrist, obstetrician, paediatrician or GP—need to balance the benefits of taking medication against any risks it may present, as virtually all medications taken by the mother will cross the placenta and be present in breastmilk. The appendix provides an overview of the safety of psychotropic medications during pregnancy.

A traumatic labour and delivery

Impregnable: A woman whose memory of labour is still vivid.

Anon.

A dramatic labour and delivery can leave a lasting imprint. Most women trust they'll have a birthing experience that is at least partly under their control. Ideally, the obstetrician will have asked the mother-to-be what she would like to have happen at the birth and will respect her preferences as much as possible. Such preferences can, however, be eclipsed by the circumstances of the birth; the process can be unpredictable and medical intervention can quickly become necessary in the face of escalating difficulties.

If the birth has been very challenging and/or the woman has experienced it as traumatic, she may later suffer flashbacks, reliving the birth. In severe cases these women qualify for a diagnosis of post-traumatic stress disorder (PTSD). The possibility of PTSD is often overlooked by diagnosing health professionals and the symptoms can be misinterpreted as PND. The key to PTSD is how stressful the labour was for the mother and may be unrelated to the *type* of delivery. If your birth plans go awry, it can be extremely helpful to discuss them and their consequences with a professional who is familiar with your circumstances. Sophia provides a typical example:

> Our 'little baby boy' wasn't exactly little, weighing in at 11 pounds [5 kilograms] after a natural birth with no drugs. They say you forget the pain. Not when your baby is already two months old when he is born! I relived that pain every day for weeks and weeks and was put off childbirth forever.

Another concern, and a focus of rumination for women who are disappointed with how the birth turned out, is that they feel they haven't done the best by their baby. Airing such preoccupations to someone she trusts can help a new mother put distressing experiences into perspective. We suggest that by expressing her fears and feelings she can release the energy bound up in regret and redirect it to nurturing her baby—and herself. Skip the phrase 'If only . . .'

Psychological risk factors

Psychological risk factors include aspects of temperament, personality and coping styles. Some are influenced by how the woman herself was parented. Psychological risk factors may compromise our ability to deploy our inbuilt protective mechanisms such as resilience, endurance and resourcefulness.

A WORD ABOUT RUMINATION

Chewing over your problems too much just makes them harder to swallow.

Anon.

Rumination (or brooding)—the process of continually mulling things over—can be very disabling and has been described as 'problem-solving gone awry'. There is a neurobiological basis to this constant looping of grim thoughts. Women with depression are more likely to fall into repetitive and circular negative thought patterns featuring guilt, blame and self-criticism. Rumination is a significant risk factor for developing a perinatal mood disorder: those who ruminate are not only more likely to become depressed but also to stay depressed. Effective techniques, such as cognitive behavioural therapy (CBT), are available for lifting yourself out of this cycle of oppressive (and obsessive) thoughts. Seek help by talking first to your GP.

The childhood experience of being parented

Mirror, mirror on the wall, I am my mother after all.

Anon.

The way in which we experience being cared for when we were children lays the foundation for our patterns of relating to other people throughout our life. Our innate temperament, which is determined by genetic mix, provides the bedrock or hardwiring—so we may be inherently set to optimism or shyness or to showing other personality traits. Having said that, we form our attitudes about ourselves, about relationships in general and about parent–child relationships in particular on the basis of early bonding experiences, most intimately with our parents but also with other stable and enduring figures, such as our grandparents, aunts, uncles, siblings. Our own parents can become our role models for parenting, whether positive or negative, as Susan testifies:

*My mother had always told us how hard it was when we were little,
how she had been miserable, how tired she always was. She was angry
and resentful—all our life. We seldom felt wanted or loved.*

At the negative end of the spectrum, being unwanted, unloved or
subjected to noxious levels of criticism, hostility or rejection, an overly
protective style of parenting or the absence of a parent can also influence
our adjustment to becoming a parent. The consequences of this type
of upbringing, such as low self-esteem, insecurity, social reserve and
pessimism, can increase the risk of developing PND and make adjustment to parenting your own offspring more stressful and complex.

Even if one or both new parents have come from psychologically
damaging backgrounds, they can modify that blueprint by choice
and circumstance, with advice and support, and thus initiate a
positive cycle for their own interactions with their children. The
blueprint handed down from one generation to the next typically
supports 'good enough' parenting, which most people find achievable and which produces well-adjusted children.

Daughters becoming mothers

A Freudian slip: when you say one thing and mean your mother.

Anon.

Many young mothers starting out as parents are determined to be a
different mother from their own (in shorthand, a 'better' one). This
sets them on a bumpier road. First, they are *reacting* to past experience—investing energy in *not* reproducing their own experience of
being parented. This distracts them from *acting*, or making a definite
attempt to do what they want to do. Additionally, most people find it
hard to create a style of mothering they have not experienced.

For a new mother on a mission to become an ideal parent, it
is easy to overshoot and aim too high. She will have no frame of
reference for the 'ideal', and so have a constant sense that she might
not be achieving it. There are two balms for this constant chafing.
First, she can try to understand and forgive the mistakes her parents

made and get them into perspective. Were they so bad? If so, were there understandable circumstances, strains or hardships? Were their intentions good at least? She could select what she *did* like and use these aspects, and discard her disappointments as much as possible. This may set a fresh baseline, allow her to be kinder to and less demanding of herself, and free her up enough to become a more typical parent. The baby is not just impressionable putty, and it takes a pretty high and constant level of abuse to have a marked negative effect on infant psychological development.

Personality style

Personality is the combination of qualities, style of social interaction and behaviours that reflect our individual nature or character (in other words, our temperament) modified by the developmental factors we face. For most people, their personality is dynamic in that they adjust their interaction with others as appropriate. Those with personality disorders, however, tend to have inflexible and rigid personality styles that do not change according to their circumstances.

As outlined below, some personality styles can increase the risk of developing depression during pregnancy and after childbirth, particularly if compounded by stressors (such as a sick baby, moving house, financial pressures). Our personality style also influences how we process information (is the glass half empty or half full?) and shapes our perception of the world.

Here we consider the influence of four common personality styles that can increase the risk of developing non-melancholic depressive conditions (see Chapter 1) during the perinatal period: socially avoidant tendencies, self-criticism, anxiousness and perfectionism. Personality styles are less relevant risk factors for the more biological illnesses: melancholic, bipolar and puerperal psychotic depression (see Chapter 1), although personality style may influence their impact on the course of the illness.

SOCIALLY AVOIDANT TENDENCIES

A woman who is socially avoidant (or excessively shy) lacks self-confidence, doesn't mix much, tends to stay at home and often spends a lot of time alone with the baby. Her thought patterns might be, 'People will be looking at me and judging me if I go out in public with the baby. Nobody talks to me when I do go out. I don't know what to say when someone strikes up a conversation. It's easier to stay home and not disrupt the baby's routines . . .' Her self-doubts feed on each other and her social isolation ensures that she avoids others, even though they could provide advice and support. If she develops depression, her tendency is to keep such pain to herself, and to be distrustful about telling others and reluctant to take up most recommended treatment options.

SELF-CRITICISM

People with self-critical traits have ongoing low self-esteem, feel inferior and often have difficulty accepting positive input from others. The thought patterns of mothers with these traits include, 'I'm not good at this. Everyone else seems so organised and in control when I see them out with their babies. I feel so inadequate.' These attitudes put them at a distinct risk of developing depression (in which their self-esteem drops even lower) and also corrode their ability to take credit for their mothering successes. They don't register their successes but only note perceived failures and mistakes.

ANXIOUSNESS

A woman with a tendency to be an anxious worrier feels apprehensive a lot of the time and, as a mother, often focuses her concerns around her own perceived limitations or her baby's health and behaviour. Such women can be difficult to reassure and are generally pessimistic. As a new mother she might find it difficult to sleep because of worry (is the baby too hot, too cold, still breathing?). She is constantly vigilant. During the day she is unlikely to unwind as the competition between trying to manage household tasks and attend to the baby bothers her and makes her feel guilty and inadequate. Such mothers tend to be overprotective of their babies and children and over-concerned about risks to safety and security.

Women who have already been diagnosed with generalised anxiety, panic attacks or obsessive compulsive disorder (OCD) are also more likely to have difficulties during pregnancy and run an increased risk of developing PND. Those with OCD may have distressing obsessions (such as the worry they might drop or otherwise harm their baby) that are completely out of character with their true caring instincts, and are never acted upon.

In her essay, Emily described a long history of mental-health-related issues and an obsessional and anxious personality pattern that she recognised as contributing to her perinatal problems. At 16 she had developed anorexia, leading to years of anguish for her and her family. When her food and body image issues were resolved, obsessive compulsive and anxiety disorders emerged more overtly:

After our honeymoon I was desperate for a baby and, while my husband wanted children, I feel he was rushed into it. Our first positive pregnancy test was a bittersweet moment. I had some problems and given my tendency to 'all or nothing' thinking was sure I would miscarry. Despite problems lasting several weeks, tests revealed a normal pregnancy. My thought patterns were not so normal. Instead of reading about baby care and nursery furniture, I googled 'pregnancy complications' over and over. Retaining my job was difficult as my work was often interrupted with internet searches in a bid to allay my fears.

Assurance came in the form of monthly appointments, which mapped a healthy heartbeat and increasing foetal growth. But, as is the case with an anxiety disorder, any assurance was short-lived. At each appointment I would present a full typed A4 document to my GP, detailing my many concerns. My anxiety reached epic proportions at 36 weeks gestation when my abdominal measurements were stagnant. A week later I developed shingles from the stress. But despite a concerning pregnancy, our healthy baby was born a week past his due date and perfect in every way.

Two weeks of bliss followed. Our baby and motherhood were everything I'd hoped and dreamed. But then Billy started to cry for hours on end, stayed awake around the clock and demanded my constant attention.

My husband, who was working away from Monday to Thursday, could do no right. When he helped, he did it wrong; when he didn't, he was no support. I can't blame him for withdrawing. I enlisted the help of sleep school, websites and countless books, not to mention unsolicited advice from strangers, but still felt like I was failing at my most important task and losing myself in the process.

So I made contact with our early motherhood service professional. Her stay was short and she assured me I had no issues besides the normal adjustment difficulties. I suppose deep down I knew better, but at the time that's what I wanted to hear. And so my anxiety continued to bubble under the surface.

Life, thank goodness, marches on. Things improved for our family. My husband entered into a local business partnership, which brought him home. His support and his presence as another adult in the house to provide intellectual stimulation and companionship helped immensely. And while I'm angry that anxiety complicated this joyous time, according to my husband the worst was yet to come. For him, the pregnancy with our second child was the hardest time in our marriage.

When Billy was 15 months old we decided to try again and, while it took only two months to conceive, I miscarried. I was devastated and irrationally scared that we would never have another child. My husband, though also feeling our loss, remained level-headed. He reasoned that miscarriages are common and another healthy baby would come along soon enough. And so it did . . . I fell pregnant soon after.

But my anxieties had increased since our first pregnancy. The miscarriage had proved to me that things can and do go wrong. With each trimester of this pregnancy came a host of fears—listeria, toxoplasmosis, chromosomal abnormalities, heart defects, pre-eclampsia, gestational diabetes, preterm labour, group B streptococcus infection, stillbirth . . . my list went on and on. The anxieties in my head were like suitcases on a conveyer belt . . . one fell off merely to make room for another.

My husband, a divine cook and great lover of fine cuisine, struggled. Meat had to be charred to a point of unpalatable dryness, vegetables washed and rewashed. I monitored the temperature of our refrigerator obsessively. Most of the time my husband put up with the fuss and caved in to my ridiculous demands, but at times it wore him down. Teamed with long hours running his own business, a wife teetering on the edge of depression was nearly too much. But he stuck by me, picked his battles and decided that some things weren't worth challenging. Also, from his earlier experience he knew that pregnancy was the worst time and the end was in sight; and though he didn't expect my obsessions to go away overnight, he knew it would be different after we had our baby.

And it was different when Ted arrived, but there were still issues and, despite a low-risk score on the Edinburgh Test [see Chapter 3], I once again contacted the early motherhood service. This time I saw a really compatible woman and had eight months of counselling and cognitive behavioural therapy. My husband attended a session and was enlightened when she explained the complexities of my condition. As I became reacquainted with myself, I realised there were trends: for each pregnancy there was one major anxiety, accompanied by a plethora of sub-anxieties. She taught me deep breathing, distraction exercises and how to challenge my thoughts, and gave me exposure therapy that prevented possible agoraphobia.

My husband laughs as he remembers thinking he would prefer celibacy to another pregnancy, following our traumatic time with Ted. But when Kristy arrived, we felt truly blessed—our third perfect child. And this time we had done it together.

My advice? Contact a counsellor—it's very important that it's someone you connect with—strengthen relationships with family, particularly your partner, and take regular physical activity.

PERFECTIONISM

I didn't want my baby picking up on my negative emotions so I used all my strength and determination to portray feelings of a happy and competent new mother and this is what I became. The house sparkled, my baby sparkled but I diminished.

Michaela

Many women are driven to maintain high standards of order and cleanliness, seeking control and order. Such mothers are likely to find the lack of clear patterns and routines associated with parenting quite challenging and stressful. They tend to be stoic and put on a brave front. They ensure they are well groomed. They often believe they are unique in their depression. They say, 'All the other mothers I see seem to be coping.' It's worth asking the question in return: 'What would other mothers see if they saw you?'

Michaela describes how her perfectionist personality contributed to every stage of her pregnancy and her postnatal experience, fuelling high stress levels. It took Michaela two years to conceive, with her husband suffering through every one of those 24 months and supporting her through the tears, the questioning and the recording of temperatures. When at last she became pregnant, she was euphoric. She welcomed the morning sickness: it was an acknowledgment of a healthy pregnancy. She felt her mission was 'to procreate, to process, to produce'. Her pregnancy was a breeze: 'I felt fulfilled, saint-like.'

Michaela continues:

By now you may have realised that my nature tends to perfectionism! The perfect pregnancy, the perfect baby, the perfect mother. My baby daughter was delivered into a quiet delivery room with low lights and little resistance from me. Her journey into the world was a silent one without cries of pain or trauma. Silence. She was whisked away and returned to me with an acknowledgment, that yes, she was indeed the perfect child; a rating of nine on the Apgar scale.

My daughter's large, gentle eyes regarded me with such trust. She looked at me with the expectation that I would take control, but after wiping away the tears of emotion, something extraordinary happened. I realised I was not prepared for the responsibility of leading her through childhood and into adulthood. I was exhausted, mentally and physically. I wanted to be mothered, not to mother. In the early hours of the morning, in a private hospital ward, I found myself alone with this newborn. I was tired, exhausted. Sleep eluded me.

The ensuing days were difficult. I prepared myself for visiting hours, making sure my daughter was fed and asleep long before family and friends arrived. Not one visitor experienced the warmth and delicious scent of my newborn; she was safely cocooned in her crib beside my bed. Perfection. But the physical and emotional roller-coaster I was on was frightening. Outwardly I appeared in control. This is as it should be. A loving mother, a competent mother, a perfect child. Oh, where was my own mother? I felt childlike, I needed her to caress my forehead and tell me she would take care of me. I felt quite alone. What if I got it wrong?

It was time to take my precious daughter home. She was perfect. I was not. The cracks would soon begin to show. I was broken. But I took to the role of motherhood perfectly. 'You're very confident. How do you know what to do?' my husband would ask. 'Instinct,' I would reply. My husband was unaware of my suffering and inner turmoil. I was functioning, that was all that mattered. The baby was thriving, that was all that mattered. Meals were on the table, the house was pristine, that was all that mattered. Outwardly, I smiled, I functioned. Inwardly, I felt nothing, I became zombie-like. No feelings. It was as if my baby had taken part of me when she slipped into the world and left this shell of a woman behind.

Eventually I sought help from the early childhood clinic during an appointment to discuss my daughter's progress. I was asked how I was coping and for once I answered honestly when I realised I could bear it no longer. A home nurse was sent to the house with pamphlets. I read them and left them on the coffee table for my husband to read. He didn't notice them and they remained unread. I was paralysed when it came to discussing my feelings or asking for help, especially from friends or family. It was the shame, you see, the feeling of not being able to cope mentally. Me, not a hair out of place, the capable one, surely not.

In describing her first few weeks at home with her new daughter, Minnie demonstrates anxiousness, along with elements of perfectionism. When her husband came home from work and asked what was for dinner, she couldn't tell him—she didn't even know how she'd managed to get dressed, let alone how she would be able to plan and produce a meal:

I couldn't leave the house. It was just too much to even consider. The thoughts in my head would race at the very idea. Even just a walk around the neighbourhood would make me feel sick. What do I need to take? Two changes of clothes, four nappies, wipes, cloth nappies for chuck, hat, toys, keys, phone, money. Have to get dressed. What's the temperature? How many layers should I put on Amy? How many layers should I put on myself? Do I need the cocoon, sunshade or rain cover for the pram? Where is the pram? Keys—need keys to get pram out of car—now where did I put the keys? Nappy bag, get keys . . . Why did I need the keys? Oh, that's right, pram!

Should I wear runners or will sneakers do? Oh no, she seems tired. Should I still go? What if she falls asleep? How will I get her back in the house? Will I leave her in the pram and try to get the pram up the four steep steps? Or take her out first? What if she wakes while I'm taking her out of the pram? Does that mean I have to feed her again? But I might not have enough milk by then and then her next feed will be early . . . Can I stretch that out so I don't muck up the routine, because if she wakes and I feed her early then she'll wake early again and she'll scream during her bath because she'll be hungry? Can I handle that? But if I feed her before the bath she probably won't go to sleep. Maybe I could do one side first, then the other after the bath? But then she'll wake in the night because she didn't get her last full feed immediately before bed. No, she's too tired: I'll put her to bed now.

All those thoughts just for a walk. How on earth could I cook dinner? I didn't have an appetite. How could I even go to the shops? I was exhausted! Amy was, as my friend would say, an unusually easy baby. She fed, burped, played, slept like clockwork; she even started sleeping 12-hour nights from three months. I thought I had no right to feel like this. I had it easy. What was my problem? Why couldn't I do a simple thing like go for a walk, prepare dinner and do a load of washing without Rick having to tell me he didn't have any undies left or a towel to dry himself after a shower?

Finally I started seeing a counsellor once a fortnight. She 'got' me. She understood everything and the thought processes that were happening in my head. After a while of me just talking, she suggested techniques to help wind down my thoughts so I could relax. I never felt pressured to try anything she suggested. One day she brought over some cards with different emotions written on them and asked me to put them into piles of how I felt, would like to feel and what didn't relate to me. It was fantastic—we discussed each card: why I felt each emotion, and the cards I wanted to feel. I could now see some of the reasons for my feelings—it was all starting to make sense.

I borrowed the cards. Rick and I had also been going through a rough patch. This was taking its toll on him, too, and I wanted to try and explain some of my thoughts so he could understand some of my actions. I couldn't believe he agreed to do it. We sat on the floor with some wine and the emotion cards and by the end of the night we were exhausted from talking and me crying, and we made some sense of how we felt and why. We understood each other better than ever and made some plans to rid ourselves of certain emotions and get back the ones we wanted.

Over the months my counsellor couldn't believe the change in me and in my relationship with Rick. I was a different person. I had confidence and I was happy and I was finally enjoying my daughter.

Social risk factors

An older mother, of multiples, born prematurely in a difficult birth, and a history of depression. On paper, I was almost guaranteed to suffer postnatal depression. But we don't live on paper, do we?

Ivana

As we considered in Chapter 1, 'stressor' is the name given to a situation or an environment that is generally experienced as unpleasant and that causes strain. Stressors can be from the past or recent and acute (short-term), chronic (long-term) or acute-on-chronic (flaring up repeatedly). The risk factors that lower our resistance to low mood and anxiety are most often an interaction between stressful events and our individual susceptibilities and personality style.

Important stressors during the perinatal period include:

- *Past (distal) stressors*, ranging from a childhood background of deprivation—be it neglect or abuse—experienced by the mother herself, to issues in previous pregnancies, such as a stillbirth, miscarriage or termination.
- *Recent (proximal) stressors*, including difficulties during pregnancy, problems in the woman's relationship with her partner, absence of a partner, lack of a supportive family or friends, housing problems, geographic isolation, too much or too little advice, the over-rosy media depiction of motherhood, other mothers' attitudes (both good and bad), and lack of sleep—this last is a very significant stressor.
- *Delivery-related stressors*, including a premature birth or an ill baby, an emergency delivery, and a long and painful labour. Lack of practical support following the baby's birth is a common stressor—both psychologically and in not allowing the mother the necessary rest and time to spend with her new baby—and is a heightened risk factor when the baby is unable to settle into feeding and sleeping.
- *Other stressors*, including whether it is a multiple birth, the baby's temperament (especially those who do not settle) and the rivalries and problems thrown up by other children in the family.
- *Chronic (long-term) stressors* can come into play, too, including dealing with work demands, being a single parent and the challenges of a blended family.

Social support

There are different types of social support.

- *Practical or 'instrumental' support*, a lack of which is a significant risk factor for PND. It can be subdivided into baby-related and household-related help.
- *Emotional support*, which allows women to be able to speak with support networks about the trials and tribulations—as well as the joys—of being a mother. It's colloquially known as 'having a shoulder to cry on'. Absence of emotional support is

also a strong risk factor for PND. All research findings highlight that lack of support from the woman's partner is one of the most potent risk factors for PND.

- *Knowledge support*, which allows women to gain information about looking after their baby. It often comes from older women, such as their own mother and mother-in-law. It could be described as the 'wisdom of the elders'. Sometimes, however, the knowledge provided via these sources can be incorrect or outdated. It is important to find the *right* person from whom to seek information.

Personal experience of social risk factors

The women's stories that follow illustrate some social risk factors: an unwanted abortion, isolation and lack of support, the tension of bridging two cultures, preparing for a disabled baby and the challenge of twins.

AN UNWANTED ABORTION

Lorraine was 21 with a 2-year-old daughter and another just 6 months old when she became pregnant again. She observed that she was not a single mum but 'might as well have been', as her partner worked away on oil rigs for months at a time. Despite having to do it all herself, she loved being a mum; her children were her friends and they spent all day, every day together.

She rang her partner, Sam, to share the news:

Perhaps it would be a boy this time and Sam would be happy, I thought.

I remember the phone call, muffled and difficult to hear as he was hundreds of kilometres out at sea. I told him the news and his first response, without reaction, was, 'Have an abortion.' I was shocked at his sureness, disappointed and hurt that he would demand such an act from me. I hung up the phone with a terrible guilt for what I was about to do. My heart was bleeding with sadness but my head ached with the thought that it was best for everyone.

My mum rang the next day from interstate and I told her the news. I could tell straight away that she thought I was a fool to let this happen only months after giving birth to my second daughter. She voiced her concerns for my wellbeing and firmly insisted that an abortion was the right thing to do. I remembered feeling confused, anxious and not sure if I was doing the right thing, but no one was saying I should keep the baby. I felt alone with no support, hurt and guilty that there was no compassion for my unborn child, and a terrible lack of confidence as a mother in an eroding relationship.

The clinic was cold and sterile, the nurses stern and regimented as they directed me to take off my clothes and put on this white gown. My name was called out and I was herded like a cow down this long corridor to the operating room. The nurse was blunt to the point of rudeness as she directed with a nod of her head to climb up onto the table where she proceeded to strap my legs to stirrups. I felt ashamed, full of guilt and like the scum of the earth. Counting down from ten, it was not long before I was out.

I woke groggy and disoriented to a nurse prodding me and saying, 'You can't sleep all day. Come on, up you get.' My friend was there, waiting to collect me. I was in no state to drive home or care for myself. I stayed the night at her place and slept most of the next day. It was over and now I just had to get on with life. I went home and took up my routine as usual but I felt empty. I pushed myself through each day with a sunken heart.

My partner was meant to come home that month but decided to save the airfare back to Perth and stay in Darwin where he had family. I understood his actions but somehow I had this gut-wrenching feeling there was more to him not returning than he let on. I was in this deep dark hole, sinking further down each day, with no thoughts of how to get out. I couldn't feel good about anything. I tried to play with the girls but it was hard pretending to be happy. Life was too much of an effort, life was lonely, life was sad. I just wanted peace and happiness again.

I started to think about death. It was as though death was the way out I knew how to take. Death did not seem so bad, in fact the thought of death felt wonderful as I would be free of all the sadness I carried. But what about my children? There was no one who could look after them as well as me, and what a terrible mother I would be if I left them here to have to endure the sufferings of life on earth all alone. If I was to go I would take them with me, of that I was sure, as I loved them dearly.

I did not realise at the time that my thoughts were irrational. I did not realise that I was planning to commit a crime so horrible that my thoughts of it today implode my world. Depression was something that was never talked about. But lucky for us all my friend was all too well aware of depression and the years of suffering her father endured before ending it. My friend told me that much research had happened since then and neurologists know that the brain is wired to live. For our brain to think that death is an option would clearly indicate an imbalance of chemicals. If the imbalance is rectified the thoughts of death disappear and rational thought is regained. She talked of levels of imbalance where sometimes it was simply a matter of talking issues through with someone, exercise and increased vitamin intake to balance the brain. Other times a doctor would need to be consulted.

That afternoon my mum rang to see how I was. I told her how I was feeling. She said there was no point sitting around crying or feeling sad—'Where's that going to get you?' And although those words brought me little comfort, she did say one thing that got me thinking: 'It's not like you to let anyone get you down. Go on, get up and fight for what you want.' Her words were stern and they made an impact. The words from my friend and the encouragement from my mother gave me enough strength to recognise that my mind was not thinking rationally and that there was no way I was going to let other people's judgements or actions stop me from having the best life I could have. I then found my strength and it came from knowledge about depression and support from family. For me I found that positive thoughts, taking multivitamins and extra B vitamins, and getting some exercise made a big difference, and I got back to myself.

It has been 27 years since the day I was so low. I went on to have two more beautiful children, one a son, and then I completed a degree at university. Next I worked in real estate and now I can sit back and enjoy the results from the labours of my life and the pleasure of my first grandchild.

Life really can be beautiful if you give it a chance.

ISOLATION AND LACK OF SUPPORT

> *It was like sinking rapidly into a thick, damp fog that I could not see through in any direction—completely unexpected and confronting. Why did I allow myself to wallow in it for so long before I finally admitted I needed help?*
>
> Nadia

Nadia was aware what kindled her depression: isolation and loneliness provided the fuel. Although she was isolated geographically from family and friends, she was also isolated emotionally from any like-minded maternal community. She was 'beyond lonely' in a new house with only an unhappy infant for hours and 'a market of baby-care books that provided useless, empty promises'. She observed that her infant daughter was not the baby the books described—she did not sleep according to the detailed charts or breastfeed according to the timetables. She abhorred being alone. Instead, she cried. 'Often. Loudly. Insistently.' Nadia held her and often cried along with her.

She described what it was like:

> *Just over four years ago my husband and I moved to a new city, far from any family or friends. Two weeks later I discovered to my surprise that I was pregnant. I suffered through the early months of my pregnancy, loneliness and anxiety exacerbated by all-day morning sickness. Usually a career-focused person, I suddenly found myself hurtling toward the realm of not working. Worried about the perceptions of others, I fiercely judged the direction my life was taking and questioned my value to society.*
>
> *Medically, my pregnancy was relatively uneventful. I underwent the standard checks and tests, all with the dutiful emphasis on finding something 'wrong'. Medical personnel were busy and distracted. I was just another pregnant woman. My labour was socially and culturally acceptable to them—hours of contractions followed by an epidural, finally finished with a vacuum-assisted delivery. The baby was out. But she cried and she cried. For hours each day.*

Leaving her to cry alone felt physically wrong. She liked to breast-feed whenever she wanted. She liked to be held. I did not want to be away from her—I just wanted to feel all right. Why were people telling me that the only way to heal myself was to ignore my baby? I did not need ephemeral baby-care solutions—I just needed nurturance as a mother.

With my husband working long shifts, there were days when I believed I could not have even five minutes to myself to eat, shower or brush my hair. Slowly, I found myself sinking.

In her essay titled 'Overwhelmed', Eleni also portrayed the impact of lack of support. While many women with perinatal depression *internalise* their depression—that is, withdraw and cry—a significant percentage *externalise* it, through irritability and anger, which is often quite uncharacteristic of their general behaviour. Predictably they then experience guilt and shame. Eleni takes us into her world—where she is clearly shocked by her own behaviour. She had never previously thought that her mental health was a problem. Occasionally when younger she'd have down times, wouldn't speak to anyone for a week and would 'revel in listening to cheesy eighties music and writing bad poetry'. As a young single woman, being occasionally mildly depressed was par for the course:

That was before I had kids.

Recently I had my second child, a gorgeous girl who, unlike her brother, finds the world a frustrating and stressful place. She communicates with unhappy screaming a lot of the time. When she's happy though, the whole world smiles with her . . . it's just that these times are few and far between.

As I write this I am aware that I am still recovering from the 'episode', as I call it. I still think about the relationship between my baby and me with reservation. I fear if I tell people I am doing better, they'll think I'm lying, because isn't that what depressed people do?

There was a particularly stressful two-week period where she was rarely happy. I was drowning in a sea of unhappiness. I just couldn't see the light and my anger was being directed at my children, albeit verbally. At this point I was simply the grumpy mum—until something or possibly nothing tipped me over the edge.

My daughter's constant screaming had set into my shoulder blades, making me feel as though I was being simultaneously crushed and stretched from the neck down. As bedtime approached I would feel unbearably anxious. I completely dreaded bedtime and there were at least four of them every day.

This day I approached my daughter's cot after trying to settle her for most of the afternoon. I'd been doing all the right things: talking soothingly, rocking and shushing. I was already emotionally fraught. After a particularly poignant wail I leaned over her cot, engaged her in direct eye contact, and said, in a flat voice, 'Shut up or I will kill you.' Then I smacked her cheek. She was 4 months old.

I want to be honest with you because no one was honest with me. If they were, I might have felt as though my feelings of anger, stress, isolation and violence were, though not acceptable . . . at least normal. I might have felt safe to tell others how I was feeling. Instead, I immediately saw my actions as proof of what I (and probably many of us) think about ourselves in the deepest darkest corners of our psyche—that there is something wrong with us, that we are not good and not trustworthy.

Aysha wrote about her good fortune when she finally unearthed some support that matched her needs. Her family didn't live nearby and she was too proud to ask them for help anyway. And her friends were all working full-time or didn't have children. She wrote:

So many worries! And the loneliness . . . I used to be a very social person and although I was so grateful for the time with my new little son at home and wouldn't have given it up for the world, it could be very lonely at times with just him and me.

When he was 8 weeks old I took him to a baby massage class at the hospital. Getting out of the house and to the hospital by 10 am was an effort! But this class changed my life. Not only did he love baby massage, not only was the instructor kind and considerate and made us feel that we were doing the right thing, but I met two mothers in that class whose babies were the same age as my little son. We exchanged numbers and arranged to meet for coffee.

That is what changed me. Meeting those girls was my lifeline, once a month or a fortnight or every week, whenever we had the time. Having other people going through the same things made it so much easier! To get other people's thoughts on how to approach something, or to get a hug when you needed one. We all agree that without each other we couldn't have made it through some of the difficult nights, the dark days, the rough patches.

Tansy outlines the loneliness that came with being unable to rely on her partner after the birth of their son. Soon he left her for a woman who was as childless and happy-go-lucky as she had been when they first met. Things actually improved after he left. She began to write; her baby started to walk and talk and play. They had each other, made some new friends and the town gradually got used to the two of them, just her son and her:

I can remember our first night home from hospital. It was like some weird quiz show. When the buzzer went (my baby's cry) I had to wake from my exhausted slumber and carry out a series of bizarre functions that had been shown to me in five seconds by the nurse: check nappy, fold nappy, apply nappy (don't prick the baby), pick up baby, place baby to breast. Was I depressed or just terrified?

The baby's father bought me a cheese grater instead of flowers. He rushed straight past us each visit to talk to the teenage mother in the next bed. He took photos of her and her baby. Was I depressed or just disappointed?

He went to sleep in the other room because the baby's crying woke him. The baby's crying woke me too. I spent hours standing up rocking him. My legs ached, my back ached. I constantly felt like crying. Was I depressed or just bloody exhausted?

He would come home from work. 'Why didn't you hang the washing out?' he would ask, looking at the washing in the basket underneath the clothes line. 'And what's for dinner?' He went to his studio to paint. 'I haven't had breakfast yet, or a shower,' I'd reply, but he was already gone.

If I tried to get away for an hour to walk the dogs I would come back to two cranky humans: one tiny and one old enough to know better. 'I can't handle it,' he would say. 'I can't handle the noise,' handing him over in the driveway.

I couldn't remember a time when I didn't feed him, clean him, carry him and listen for him all the time. I couldn't remember my last decent sleep. I used to think, 'I've . . . just . . . got . . . to . . . do . . . the . . . dishes . . . and . . . clean . . . my . . . teeth . . . and . . . then . . . I . . . can . . . sleep.'

I could only face the supermarket by throwing back a few swigs of neat whisky in secret. I felt like crawling into a small dark space and hiding. I felt like walking out the front gate and never, ever coming back.

We moved to a new town and I didn't know anyone. I would cart the baby around the neighbourhood trying to have a life: a walk by the beach, a visit to the markets, playgroup. I felt like a loser. His father never went anywhere with us. If he did let us go to the hardware store with him he would get out of the car and just walk off while I struggled with the car seat and the stroller, nappies and toys—all kinds of stuff I'd never needed before.

After he left and my son became a little older, I got out more. I formed strong bonds with other women in similar situations: lifetime bonds. I went to counselling and then I got a part-time job. I started playing music again and people started to visit. I was a person, not just a mother. I was a person who was also a mother.

I realised that I probably hadn't even been depressed, just the mother of a small child while living in a hopelessly inadequate relationship.

BEING CAUGHT BETWEEN CULTURES

Child rearing can be the first real exposure of a newly migrated couple to the systems and values of their adopted country. They will enter the local hospital network where the procedures for handling pregnancy, birth and postnatal follow-up are likely to be standardised for efficiency, with scant accommodation of cultural differences. Misunderstandings can arise on both sides. Limited language skills combined with isolation and the hard work needed to establish the family unit within the adoptive country add extra strain to an already challenging time for many new residents.

There may also be profound differences in the customs surrounding the perinatal period. And some families face the opposite challenge when they bring their baby home: born in Australia to migrant parents, the young parents may identify with local customs and values rather than their parents' traditions, and face conflict rather than support.

If there are mental health problems such as PND, the new mother can have difficulty accessing help, especially if her extended family lacks either understanding or acceptance of mental illness. The NSW Multicultural Health Communication Service (MHCS) provides translations of health information and guides to resources in the area; the Transcultural Mental Health Centre is also an excellent starting point.[3]

A DISABLED BABY

Shona was formally diagnosed with PND just before her first child turned 1. She did almost everything except take antidepressants, trying a myriad of non-medication therapies and couple-therapy sessions together with telephone support from PANDA (a community support organisation for sufferers of perinatal depression).

She wrote:

All these therapies were kept secret from relatives overseas. Only my friends knew and were very supportive and understanding. The fog had finally lifted after our first child's arrival. Jason was thriving and I was on the road to recovery. Then I fell pregnant with baby number two. This time I was ready. This time I was prepared.

But life threw us a curve ball.

Around 19 weeks gestation, we learnt Bronte would be born with an extra chromosome. I received the news over the phone and I was in utter shock. By sheer coincidence my mentor, Lainie, dropped by. It was through her that help came from all over: local, regional, state and national.

So long before Bronte was born, we began preparing ourselves for a unique parenting journey. We started to research as much as we could about trisomy 21 thanks to Down Syndrome Victoria⁴ and Lainie introduced me to a lactation consultant. With her help plus our fabulous midwife, Bronte was able to successfully breastfeed within minutes of being born, despite having Down syndrome, and we were sent home after a few short days. She was steadily gaining weight.

All was going well until our little girl was 8 weeks old, when she was diagnosed with a congenital heart defect: two holes in her heart that had to be fixed as soon as possible. Open-heart surgery at 12 weeks. It was a shock for all of us because she was outwardly healthy, breastfeeding, thriving and alert! No one can prepare themselves for something like this. I was fortunate to find a family doctor who takes a holistic approach to care. Asking for a script for antidepressants was my last resort, but once the medication started to work, it helped anchor me.

Our life continues its ups and downs. At the beginning, I felt that the universe had played a cruel prank on us: I shook my fists at the heavens several times. We have often asked, 'Why? Why me? Why us?'

It is a different path from what we expected and that's as much as we know. However, help is always there whenever we need it and it continues to arrive whether we seek it or not. I can't be bothered to worry now about what the future holds for us. For the present, all I can do is to enjoy the moment with my husband and children, hold them in my arms, and remember to simply breathe, breathe mindfully and take one day at a time.

UNEXPECTED ABUNDANCE: TWINS

Zara had always thought there was something special about women who had twins. They seemed to conceive easily and carried off their pregnancies with style. She was not the sort to have twins. In fact, during her first pregnancy she learned that she 'wasn't much of a breeder at all'. They had faced a desperate fight to hold onto their little daughter's life: she survived and finally thrived.

But when Zara plucked up the courage to do it all again, she found it far from easy. As miscarriage followed miscarriage, she became pessimistic. The day she first saw two minuscule hearts blipping on the ultrasound screen, her only thought was, 'How can I bear to lose two babies at once?' But she didn't lose them. While friends and family braced for a train wreck to match her first pregnancy, she blossomed. By now the 'size of a small cow', she relished the experience and the love she felt for her 4-year-old daughter and her unborn boy/girl twins seemed limitless. And then the twins were born.

Zara tells her story in 'Blessed':

In the first week home, as the happy hormones deserted my emptied-out body, I heard the drumbeats of the military campaign I should have foreseen but had not. I found myself in a boot camp of swaddling and nappies and three-hourly twin feeds that took two adults to stage-manage and one hour to complete. Within the first two weeks, I had lost the ability to sleep. The adrenaline I needed to psych myself up for the effort of each feed did not subside between sessions, so although friends and relatives gave me plenty of respite to lie down, I could not switch off. On at least two occasions, I remained awake for longer than 48 hours.

I shook with cold, I was nauseated and my thoughts became increasingly deranged. The global financial crisis was big in the news, but while my imagination took hold of the media's presentiments of doom and spun them into visions of total social collapse, all the people around me continued to behave as if life was proceeding as normal. Above me, cracks were forming in the sky, but no one else seemed to notice that it was about to fall in . . .

On one night when I did fall asleep, I woke feverish from a nightmare. 'I dreamed we had twins,' I said to my husband.

'Look in the spare room,' came an exhausted voice from under the pillow.

In the spare room, my nightmare was corporeal—two little babies, asleep in their cots. They were real. There were two of them, and they were mine. They were only weeks old, but already I was spent. I had nothing left in the tank and yet I had somehow to continue feeding them, day in, day out, from my own body. I had to clothe them, toilet train them, show them manners, read to them, earn money to educate them, teach them to drive. How was I going to do all of this when I was too exhausted to cook dinner?

At the same time as I was unhelpfully projecting myself into the distant future, I believed that the tiredness and limitations of my present condition would last forever. I felt trapped in a never-ending now that was all about dragging myself, yet again, to the couch, strapping myself into the breastfeeding pillow and attaching a pair of bottomless leeches to my breasts.

My successful career was all behind me. I knew that I would never be able to teach—read, write or think—ever again. I had lost my mind. And with me unemployed, we would be on the breadline, I told myself. My older daughter, who had experienced four years of comfort and privilege as an only child, would know that our poverty and deprivation was all my fault for wanting a second child so badly that I had produced twins and destroyed our lives.

I wasted away and hollowed out. Food repulsed me, which meant there was no way to replace the calories I was giving out. I spent a lot of time lying down, not sleeping, with catastrophic thoughts cycling through my head. If I was out of bed, I sat comatose, unable to converse.

'Just think how lucky you are,' said my mother, in an attempt to shake me out of a stupor that was frightening her. 'You have two healthy babies. You are blessed.'

The thing was, right then I didn't feel blessed. I didn't want two healthy babies. I didn't want any babies. I just wanted to go to sleep. I began to fantasise about the long, uninterrupted sleep of the drowned. I had a stretch of cliffs in mind. There were lead diving weights in the shed.

I knew I was depressed. The public discourse around postnatal depression meant that I had a strong awareness of the condition, and the rapidity with which I had plunged from 'never felt better' to 'never felt worse' made it easy for me to diagnose myself. Still, I was reluctant to seek professional help because I thought I could use my intelligence to think my way through it. I spent mornings planning my suicide and afternoons reading psychiatric textbooks.

These people kept me going: my husband, my mother, my daughter, my GP. My husband got up with me for every feed, held mugs of Milo in front of my face—with a straw—so that I could sip while I cradled a tiny skull in each of my hands. When I panicked, he insisted I bring my thoughts back from tomorrow, next week and next year, to today, this minute. Whenever I thought I might end my life, I imagined my daughter's face at the moment her father told her Mummy was never coming back.

At last, I confided in my GP, who prescribed antidepressants. I resisted. I had always seen myself as a successful, independent woman, and the blister pack of tablets in my purse seemed to rubbish all that. And yet, I knew I needed help. When I finally capitulated and took the first tablet, I felt ... nothing in particular. Gradually, though, my mind began to right itself. Slowly, I regained my aptitude for sleeping and with it my mental health.

Least helpful in my period of depression were the attitudes of health professionals I approached when I was looking for a way of getting some respite from 24-hour breastfeeding, while not giving up breastfeeding altogether. While the advice I got was wildly divergent, both sides of the argument were adamant that there was no middle ground. My obstetrician, himself a father of twins, told me I was mad to consider breastfeeding at all. Conversely, a lactation consultant—deeply entrenched in her ideology—told me I was risking my children's health with formula.

Against all advice, my husband and I worked out a system of alternating bottles and breastfeeds for each baby, allowing us to sleep in shifts. As I clocked up sleep hours, my panic and desperation subsided. The news was still full of the GFC, but the cracks in the sky no longer showed. After three months, I stopped taking medication.

My daughter is 6 now and my twins are 2—bonny and bumptious. I have made it back to work, where I find that I can teach and write and read and think after all. Life is busy and tiring, but not unmanageably so.

The other day, I was running through town in the rain with my twins. We took shelter under a shop awning, all three of us laughing as we shook the raindrops off our faces. For an instant, I caught our reflection in a shop window—a happy mother with matching toddlers, one holding each hand.

And so it turns out that I am *blessed after all.*

SUMMARY

This chapter has provided an overview of the biological, psychological and social risk factors that can act as primary and secondary causes of PND, and the quite variable contexts and ways that PND is experienced and addressed. Becoming aware of the risk factors that can increase your vulnerability to PND will enable you to marshal pre-emptive strategies. A competent assessment of any postnatal disorder by a health professional should determine the principal and contributing causes in order to derive an effective management plan. Any such plan should also respect the woman's own story and world view.

three

Screening for
perinatal depression

The thoughts of two health professionals about picking up on perinatal mood problems:

'I'm not saying I actively look for it, but I am hoping my antennae would tell me if there was a problem.'

'I think any kind of flatness . . . it's a difficult thing to explain, isn't it? . . . You can just tell by having a conversation . . . just chatting to them.'[1]

The tools we use to screen for PND don't diagnose depression but identify women who may need referral for further evaluation and diagnostic clarification. Screening is akin to a mammogram—it is not definitive but broadly indicates either an all clear or a concern that requires further investigation.

One complication of screening is, paradoxically, the woman herself. Women with a postnatal mood condition often fear being labelled with the diagnosis and what they think will be its consequences—including separation from their baby. In response, many struggle on, avoiding any help and keeping their mask ('I'm loving it!') firmly in place. Even the most skilled health professional can miss PND, especially if the woman isn't giving clear or honest indications of how she is feeling.

beyondblue, Australia's national depression initiative, provides excellent information on its website, particularly via its 'beyond babyblues' program.[2]

A HEALTHCARE WORKER'S TACT UNCOVERS A PROBLEM

Jacinta returned to Australia after a heady two-year stint in London where she and her husband had worked hard, earned well and enjoyed life. Two months after her return she gave birth. In her unfamiliar new house with her colicky baby she felt that she had suddenly migrated to a different planet. Each day she struggled to avert overwhelming mess: binfuls of soiled nappies, an empty fridge, a full sink, a white floor she couldn't keep clean, days when there was nowhere to walk but the strange dark rooms of their new house. When she finally made it out into daylight, her 3-week-old baby would come crying with her and they 'would disturb everyone else's peace'.

By her son's sixth month, she was averaging two to four hours' sleep per night. One early morning her weariness was so great that to move from one room to another she crawled across the floor. She finally began to ask herself was she simply sleep-deprived or was a pervading sadness affecting her sleep and ability to cope?

It was her maternal health nurse's understanding and recommendations that pushed Jacinta towards recovery. Jacinta names her two stumbling blocks: initially, non-recognition of her depression and next, her unwillingness to brave the stigma that might come with the label of PND.

She continues:

Given that before I'd left for London and my new life two years previously I had interviewed and written about one of mental health's greatest Australian ambassadors, Neil Cole, I should have recognised my symptoms and acted upon them. But how does one know if the mood that has descended is what is to be expected for someone mourning the death of a particular lifestyle—or postnatal depression?

I should have seen the signs and acted on them. I didn't. I was tested only because this was part of my maternal health nurse's routine. She was careful and casual in the way that she handed me the questionnaire. I am still thankful for her sensitivity.

Perhaps I understood too well the repercussions of 'coming out'. I didn't want anyone outside of my partner and mother to know how troubled I was, so whenever an answer wasn't clear and I could choose one multiple choice over another, I ticked the more lenient option. My test results confirmed the verdict: I was on the borderline of postnatal depression.

In his memoir about depression, Never Real and Always True, *James Bradley describes his liberation at knowing that the thing that afflicted him had a name. Neil Cole has also spoken of relief in receiving his bipolar disorder diagnosis. As much as I applaud their honesty and courage, I could never be that open or brave, but I did seek help and it was of inestimable benefit, though it took me some time to find the right fit for my maladies.*

And what about the stigma that prevented me from looking for support once I recognised my depression? Positive changes in society's perception will occur only when we begin to see mental health as part of a continuum we are all on. In other words, if it doesn't hurt to wear the label, more people might be prepared to wear it.

A woman's difficulties can be alleviated without labelling her, however, and she might more readily look for help if she knows what the consequences might be. We'll now briefly consider some screening measures: one that covers the perinatal period (the two-question screen), one that assesses a woman's risk of developing PND (the antenatal risk questionnaire), and a measure that aims to identify current PND. At the end of this chapter, we outline the various care pathways and where they might lead.

SCREENING TOOLS FOR PND

The two-question screen

The two-question screen[3] is a well-regarded quick screen, though not specific to the perinatal period. These two yes/no questions are asked verbally or in writing:

'During the last two weeks, have you ever been bothered by:
- feeling down, depressed, or hopeless?
- little interest or pleasure in doing things?'

Sometimes a rider is added:

• 'Is this something with which you would like help?'

If you answer yes to either question, the interviewer should follow up with further clarifying questions. An honest negative response to both questions suggests you are unlikely to be depressed.[4] While the two-question screen is brief, some have argued for an even briefer approach: enquiring about a mother's difficulty in falling asleep 'may be the most relevant screening question in relation to their risk for postpartum depression', they suggest.[5]

The antenatal risk questionnaire (ANRQ)

This measure was developed by Professor Marie-Paule Austin and colleagues in Sydney.[6] It differs from other scales in that it assesses a woman's *risk* of developing PND. It captures many of the risk factors considered earlier (see Chapter 2), including a history of mental health problems, experience of maternal deprivation, emotional or sexual abuse, previous experience of a distinct period of depression, an unsupportive partner, exposure to stressors during the preceding 12 months, lack of support, and being a worrier or perfectionistic. It was designed to be administered by trained staff and as an adjunct to a clinical interview.

The Edinburgh postnatal depression scale (EPDS)

The ten-item Edinburgh postnatal depression scale assesses the current likelihood of PND being present.[7] It asks women to score their symptoms over the past week. Four questions assess depressed mood, two anxiety, two an anhedonic mood (lack of pleasure) and non-reactive mood, one impairment, and one thoughts of self-harm.

CLINICAL SCREENING BY A HEALTH PROFESSIONAL

It should be remembered that a screening tool is just that—a quick scan to help identify possible problems. Any screening tool can generate false positives (women who score highly but who are in fact not depressed) and false negatives (failing to identify women who are clinically depressed and who would benefit from assistance).

A positive screen indicates the possibility of a diagnosis—it is *not* a diagnosis in itself.

The most accurate results from screening occur when there is an established relationship between the woman and the practitioner doing the screening. This is not always feasible: nurses might only have one contact with any particular woman. An empathic nurse, counsellor or doctor—whether a GP or a specialist who is dealing with physical difficulties in the mother or baby—can encourage a pregnant woman or new mother to open up about a depressive condition. This can happen in response to a screening tool or simply as a result of asking empathic open questions.

As Sally writes:

Within a few months of the miscarriage I was thrilled and scared to be pregnant again. When I finally arrived at my obstetrician's office 12 weeks pregnant I felt such relief. I so appreciated when he looked up from his paperwork (after noting I had had a miscarriage) and into my eyes. With compassion he said, 'So, you've had a difficult start. Let's have a look and see that baby of yours.'

This man is loved by many an expectant mother. He doesn't hide behind a mask of expertise or set himself up as the authority telling his patients what to do. This obstetrician had discovered that pregnant women need to be seen and treated as special. He knew this was more than a physical, medical event. Much of the time pregnant women are expected to just continue on as always with the only—inadequate— rituals to mark the transition to mother being antenatal classes and a baby shower.

Empathic questions

Skill is needed in establishing trust and creating an environment that feels safe. Some interviewers are able to project a sense of unhurried interest and convey non-judgemental respect. All women, even those who look as if they're coping well, and even those with older babies, deserve the benefit of screening. Women are particularly skilled at maintaining their show face, even when experiencing considerable distress. Open-ended questions (akin to those used in the interview in Chapter 4) encourage a woman to entrust the enquirer with her experience.

Open-ended empathic questions

- 'How has your pregnancy been so far? What is it like for you to be pregnant?'
- 'Often we have certain ideas about what childbirth will be like. What were your thoughts about childbirth when you were pregnant? How did that compare with what actually happened? How do you feel about the delivery when you think about it now?'
- 'Many mothers find the first few months of being a mum really hard. How are you finding it?'

If the woman expresses some distress

- 'When did you first realise that this wasn't what you expected?'
- 'What's been okay and what's not going too well?'
- 'What's it like for you, being a mum?'
- 'Having a baby often has quite an impact on relationships. Has anything been different between you and your partner since the baby came along? How is that for you? How is it for your partner?'

SCREENING IN AN OBSTETRIC HOSPITAL

Nurses sometimes skirt the subject of depression. If they have concerns or find a positive screen, it can make such a difference if they speak to the woman directly or mention it to someone who will follow it through. A mother with a positive screen is admitting to a problem and asking for help, even if unconsciously, as this story from Fiona illustrates:

When I was admitted to hospital to try and stabilise my second pregnancy, I had my first real discussion with a health professional about my experience after the birth of our first child. I still believed what I had experienced was a normal part of motherhood and that I had just handled it terribly. But these discussions began to paint a picture . . . that I had suffered a severe case of postnatal depression. I was flooded with relief to know that there were larger factors at play other than me being an appalling mother. This moment in time was like coming out of a dark cave into bright sunlight. To have a name for what I experienced and to have a medical team monitoring me for baby two had such a good effect on my perspective.

Women appreciate the following approaches from nurses and others at such a vulnerable time:

- empathising and endorsing her experience
- indicating that she is not alone, that it is a steep learning curve and that she is not to blame for any perceived lapses in her adaptation to motherhood
- emphasising that she shouldn't bury her concerns but ask for help
- indicating where she can find resources
- reassuring her that perinatal mood swings are common and that women recover from them well with assistance
- avoiding any hint of blame, especially if the mother has concerns about the potential negative effects of her condition on the development of the baby and on their bond.[8]

WHY MOTHERS OFTEN DON'T REVEAL THEIR DISTRESS

Earlier we noted some key reasons why mothers are reluctant to reveal their distress to others. These extracts give further insights:

If I had PND again, I'd approach a community health nurse. It was only after I recovered that I found they could help. The community health people seemed supportive and accepting, not judgemental. Like most human beings, I resent being managed by others, even in the name of caring.

Hannah

The things that I found unhelpful were when I went to see a different GP as my own was unavailable and I felt like I was at crisis point. This GP did not understand and I felt he really minimised my feelings. I went home feeling ashamed, uncertain and embarrassed.

Lydia

The nurse I saw for the regular check-ups following my daughter's birth showed little concern about my wellbeing after I completed a mood survey. She told me I needed to be careful as I was showing signs of depression. On my return visit, holding down a big lump in my throat, fighting back tears, I was hoping for some kind of advice . . . or even some answers, but she went ahead and did the routine check of my daughter: neither of us uttering a word about my moods. I was determined not to cry in front of her: she seemed so stoic and strong.

Lilly

It seems foolish now, but at the time I felt that if I admitted I needed help it would only make it worse. That, by bringing it out into the open, it would take on a definite (and, I feared, permanent) shape. By denying my depression it seemed as though I was able to maintain some kind of control over it. I remember at the antenatal clinic being asked to fill in a questionnaire: 'Did I feel depressed?', 'Did I feel worthless?', 'Did I lack energy?' Yes. Yes, I did. But how could I just tick a box and hand over my deepest fears, inadequacies and failings to a complete stranger? The nurses at the clinic were incredibly busy, seeing hundreds of women every week. I saw a different one every visit. How could I so casually expose myself like that? So I kept it to myself and the depression intensified after my baby was born.

Fatima

When the maternal and child health nurse suggested three months after the baby's birth that I might be suffering from postnatal depression, I rejected her suggestion with a violence that shocked me. Though I agonised about my time off work and money problems, about not being a good wife, about not being a good enough mother, about losing weight, about putting on weight, about the growing baby's health, about feeling so alone and dejected, I was besotted with my child and deter-mined to make things work, despite the lack of sleep and the swamping anxiety. But exhaustion bracketed my shrunken, colourless life.

Karla

FINDING A CARE PATHWAY

Every new mother needs reassurance that assistance is available for her and her baby should they need it. A 'care pathway' is a loose term used to describe local referral networks of support for mental health disorders of differing levels of risk, severity and complexity. A health professional can provide direction for a woman and her family so they can find the most appropriate mental health and well-being support during the perinatal period.[9] The particular pathway for a woman will depend on how much and what sort of help she is seeking, and what might provide the greatest benefit:

- For mild problems with adjustment, many community resources provide educational information, including the several websites we refer to in this book (see the 'Notes' section).
- For moderately severe mood disorders and anxiety, the GP can often provide assistance and consultation, with clinical assessment and limited mental health intervention.
- For disorders that are judged more severe again, a specialist such as a psychiatrist can assist with assessment, treatment and ongoing management.
- For severe cases, there may also be a need for acute (rapid-response) community-based mental health care or, in even more severe instances, hospital-based mental health services.[10]

Severity, however, should not be the only determinant of the care pathway and choice of health professional. A sophisticated diagnostic assessment and formulation may save years of disability by clarifying the condition and its best management, including by whom and with what resources. Thus screening is only a first stage. If a woman screens positive—or is clearly in difficulty but minimising her distress and responses to screening—the next best step is generally a detailed clinical assessment leading to a clear diagnosis.

four

Diagnosis and
treatment options

Being a mother is learning about strengths you didn't know you had,
and dealing with fears you didn't know existed.

Linda Wooten

If a woman experiences mood difficulties during her pregnancy or after her baby is born, a diagnosis (identifying the type of disorder) and a formulation (an explanation of her particular disorder in the context of contributing factors and her life story) are the best tools to classify her perinatal difficulties and to generate a management plan that will enable her to overcome them. This extract from Punita illustrates the value of a diagnosis:

I struggled with my feelings, never sure if what I was feeling was abnormal or just me. Did I have a disorder, had it all been too much for me and I was sort of ill, or was I just a lazy, disorganised, yelling and tired monster? Don't get me wrong, my house was mainly tidy, the children were fed, clean and for the most part happy, but I was a mess. My internal mess was hidden from the outside world, though, because I did not want anybody to know just how sad and horrible I felt about myself. Everybody was right. I couldn't cope so why did I have another baby? It was my fault. I had no right to complain.

Thankfully, my GP spotted my misery when I took the baby to her for his shots. She sensed my despair and although it was a shock to me initially, the diagnosis of postnatal depression gave me a name for what I was feeling and a pathway back to the 'me' that I had lost.

THE IMPACT OF A DIAGNOSIS

A diagnosis can be seen as threatening because it says there is 'something wrong'. But a diagnosis also provides relief and, strangely, reassurance. Researchers at the Black Dog Institute surveyed people who had received a diagnosis of bipolar disorder and found that many

---

WHAT IS A FORMULATION?

A formulation is more than a diagnosis. With a formulation, the assessing clinician seeks to explain *why this person* is suffering *at this particular time* with *what type of condition*. It allows for the factors that are potentially contributing to the illness to be weighed and sorted, and shapes broad management strategies into an individually tailored treatment approach.

The four Ps

A conceptual framework known as the four Ps captures the key components of a formulation:

- Protective factors—the individual's strengths, social supports and positive patterns of behaviour. These can soften the impact of stress and trauma and so contribute to resilience.
- Predisposing factors—which can set the scene and include biological and genetic causes as well as developmental stressors and experiences.
- Precipitating factors—the triggers or events that closely precede and initiate the problem, for example a change in a social situation.
- Perpetuating factors—which hinder or prevent recovery from the problem, situation or illness. For PND conditions, these factors include lack of sleep, the woman's personality style, lack of support, social isolation and an unsettled baby.

had experienced positive outcomes: the development of stronger bonds with their family, relief at finding out what was wrong and renewed purpose in achieving positive treatment outcomes. A diagnosis gave them the terminology they needed to explain their illness to others, enabled them to separate themselves from their mood disorder and feelings of guilt, and engendered optimism that their disorder could be brought under control.[1]

THE STIGMA OF A PSYCHOLOGICAL PROBLEM

When people are faced with severe or disabling *physical symptoms* they usually seek help. Depending on how intense their symptoms are and their belief about the best way to make them go away, they see their GP or another health practitioner or chat to someone. When people are faced with *psychological symptoms* they are less inclined to reach out for help, largely reflecting perceived stigma and the fact that psychological symptoms are often hard to describe and communicate. Also, the professional chosen by a woman looking for help might not display either the skills required for symptom and risk clarification, or the attitude that encourages her to reveal her private inner world and the issues central to understanding the shape of her disorder. Women also avoid asking for help if they feel they will be labelled. Their PND symptoms generally do not relate to their usual experience of normal sadness and depressed mood, and the possibility of having something wrong with them mentally is discomfiting and a threat: 'Not only am I a failure as a mother but a *nut case* as well.'

For these reasons, mothers with PND may imitate how they *should* be functioning and resist help. If they do get help, they may still express this resistance through denial and by playing down their symptoms and distress. This can distort a diagnostic assessment and any subsequent management, which is why an experienced, empathic health practitioner is vital.

Denying and minimising perinatal problems

In the extract below, from an essay titled 'One of *those* women', Pat takes us into her world and helps us understand why factors such as denial ('I'm fine') can make it so difficult to pick up the signs that a woman isn't coping. She also shows why she was unlikely to open up to any of the healthcare staff she saw.

When the nurse visited at three weeks, Pat made sure the baby was settled and the house clean so it looked like she was coping and so no one could accuse her of not doing a good job. When she took her son for his six-week check-up and was handed a survey titled 'Postnatal depression screening' she thought, 'Oh, I know what this is! Well that's not me. I'm a teacher! I'm very capable.' And so she filled out the form in the waiting room, carefully selecting options that wouldn't lead to further questioning from the midwife. 'I'm not one of those *crazy* women!' she told herself.

She was eventually able to be open about her difficulties—and in this excerpt we can observe how her self-protecting strategies of resistance and denial were influenced by her differing interactions with health professionals:

'Are you sure you're pregnant?' the midwife asks, fumbling awkwardly with her equipment. 'Yes, I'm fairly certain . . .' I say, my heart starting to race. 'Well, I can't find a heartbeat. The paperwork can't be done until we know a baby is in there. You'll need to have an ultrasound.' 'Oh, all right then . . .' I say as I am directed up the hallway. I feel numb. 'Lie down and I'll take a look,' the radiographer directs. 'I'm all alone,' I think despairingly. 'I am just about to be told there is no baby in there and I'm all alone.' Minutes pass, then I hear the radiographer's voice: 'I've found a heartbeat!' Relief! I walk back to the midwife. 'Yes, a baby is in there!' I proclaim, holding up the ultrasound. 'Good, let's get these forms filled in then,' she replies brusquely.

I continue to work full-time as a teacher. I go through my daily routine, sending the students out to recess and then shutting the blinds. I lie down in the reading corner to rest. Minutes later, the bell rings. I get up, open the door ready for class. 'How long until lunch?' I ask myself. Eventually I make it to my last day. I have taught other people's children for ten years and now I'm starting my own family. I look around at the empty classroom. I feel alone. I drive home and start to sob uncontrollably. It's hard to let go.

I have been in labour all day and the baby isn't moving. The midwife arrives to announce that my doctor has called, 'She is disappointed you haven't progressed further and suggests a caesarean.' 'Caesarean? Definitely not!' I think to myself. 'I can get this baby out if I just try a bit harder! I'm not one of those women . . .'

Hours pass and my obstetrician finally arrives to examine me. 'Your baby won't be coming out this way. Sorry,' she announces and then walks out. I begin to cry. I've failed. At 9.05 pm my son is born by emergency caesarean. He stares at me. Silently. His eyes make me nervous. 'Who are you?' I think. 'Shouldn't I instantly fall in love?' I'm exhausted. They take him away and I lie in Recovery alone. 'Where is my baby? Why are they taking so long?' I feel anxious. Finally, after an hour, they bring him down. He has been bathed. I am shocked. Shouldn't I be there for his first bath?

I have trouble with breastfeeding. The baby doesn't attach properly. My back aches and I can't move from the hospital bed. When will my milk start flowing? Why won't he attach? Why does it hurt so much? 'Stop asking so many questions. You're a mother now,' the midwife says gruffly. I go quiet. 'Silly girl! Stop asking questions. You should know what to do. You're a mother. It should come naturally,' I scold myself.

I walk inside our house with the baby. The crying begins. He won't feed, screaming all afternoon and into the night. Should I ring the hospital? I don't know what to do. He has trouble settling and hardly sleeps. He is awake sometimes for eight hours straight. He seems to cry all the time. The hospital calls after a week to see how I'm doing. 'I'm fine!' I try to sound cheery. I don't want to admit I'm finding it difficult. 'You have to remain strong!' I repeat over and over to myself.

My son is 6 weeks old and my husband is going back to work. I'm terrified. I can't be alone with the baby. Mum is coming over. She's running late. Doesn't she know I'm scared to be with the baby? When she arrives she seems confused by my lack of confidence. I wish she would just hold him so I can rest and do other things. How do you keep a baby amused all day? It's good when he is asleep. I have things to do. I need to keep this house looking clean. The baby cries and I start to feel angry. Doesn't he know I'm vacuuming? 'I'm not going to be one of those mothers with a messy house,' I remind myself.

I stand in the staffroom at work, tears streaming down my face. I'm talking to a colleague, but he ignores my emotional state. It is my first day back at work, nine months after giving birth. My mother babysits so I can work one day a week. Has anyone noticed how upset I am? I walk up to my class, holding back the tears. How am I going to stand in front of them? I'm a wreck. I can't stop thinking about my baby at home. Will Mum know what to do when he cries? I left detailed instructions about his routine and was hoping she would follow them. It is hard to focus on my job. 'A good mother would be home with her baby,' I berate myself.

My son is 13 months old and I find out I am pregnant again. I have a different obstetrician this time. I tell him how I get anxious at times. 'It's just part of my personality,' I explain. He asks if I've ever been diagnosed with anxiety or depression. 'No!' I quickly reply. 'I'm not one of those mental patients!' I think to myself.

I'm a robot. I feed my newborn baby. I change his nappy. I put him to bed. I read to my toddler. I can't wait until he's asleep. I nap for three hours. Is that the baby? I wonder how long he has been crying. Does anyone know how hard it is to look after a baby and a toddler by yourself, all day? I don't have any energy. I can't go out. I feel tense and agitated. 'But I should be able to cope . . .' I tell myself again and again.

I visit my GP for a check-up, but burst into tears. I feel embarrassed as I don't usually discuss emotional issues. 'I'm sorry,' I sob. 'I'm not doing well. I haven't been able to sleep since my first child was born. I'm exhausted.' My GP seems nervous at my display of emotion and suggests I try some warm milk and reading to help me sleep. She timidly hands me a pamphlet on pottery classes for people with anxiety. I am confused. I really want to get help but when will I find time to do pottery?

I phone a friend to chat but begin to cry uncontrollably. I am embarrassed to be revealing how I am really feeling. 'Has anyone suggested you might have postnatal depression?' she asks. 'No,' I reply defensively. My friend describes her own experience and suddenly the light switches on. Is depression really an illness? Her story sounds just like mine. She said that taking medication helped her cope. I didn't realise medication could help with how you feel.

I decide to visit another GP. I tell her that I think I have post-natal depression. She empathises and describes her experience with her own children. Relief! Finally, someone who understands. She prescribes some medication and hands me a book called Taming the Black Dog. *I cry as I read it. I don't want to feel this way anymore. Other people's experiences show me that life can be better. I take my first steps to recovery.*

Regaining my health takes longer than I expect. I try out two anti-depressants over six months before finding one that works. My doctor suggests seeing a psychologist to help with my thinking patterns. It takes a few months before I decide to make an appointment. I am surprised that I feel comfortable with her immediately. My psychologist was once a teacher. She is the mother of three teenage children. It feels like luxury to have someone who understands. The sessions help me to change my negative thought patterns and address relationship issues in my life.

With the combination of medication and therapy I have come to a place of acceptance about myself and my condition. Yes, I have postnatal depression and anxiety. Yes, I need to continue treatment to manage my condition. Yes, I had to overcome the stigma of mental illness. Yes, I am one of 'those' women—and proud to say it.

WORRIES THAT YOUR BABY WILL BE TAKEN AWAY

A powerful fear for some women is that their baby will actually be taken away if she or her partner puts up a hand to seek help for a mood disorder. The woman may panic that 'others' (such as 'services' and government departments) will gain the power to muscle in on her life if she admits to doubts about her coping.

This should reassure you: it is only in *extreme* cases of mental illness, when women don't access mental health care and are unable to care for their baby and older children, or the children are exposed to the mother's unstable mental health, or drug or alcohol abuse, that government services are called in. Even in extreme cases, child protection agencies try to ensure that the woman accesses services that will help her recover and help the family stay together.

Another fear expressed by women is that, following a marital separation, evidence of any PND might be viewed as a reason to grant custody to the father over the mother. Generally, however, a mother is much more likely to be granted custody of the baby.

HOW A HEALTH PROFESSIONAL MIGHT ASSESS A MOTHER FOR PND

The following example comes from the Black Dog Institute's training course for health professionals, entitled 'Perinatal mood disorders in practice'.[2] It illustrates a clinical approach to assessing the likelihood of PND and also to undertaking a risk assessment.

Jenny has brought her 7-week-old daughter, Ivy, to her GP. Ivy has been crying inconsolably for hours every afternoon. Her GP has completed a history and examination of the baby and is unable to find any underlying cause for the prolonged crying.

Most of the clinician's questions are open, encouraging Jenny to respond expansively, rather than closed questions with yes/no answers. A skilled clinical interview generally mixes both types of question, as can be observed in the example below. The interviewer's empathic attitude is also evident and is central to the success of the interview, advancing mutual respect and trust.

INTERVIEW BETWEEN JENNY AND HER GP, FOLLOWING IVY'S EXAMINATION

GP: It can be very challenging having a baby that cries for such long stretches. A lot of mothers would find it distressing and hard to cope with. How are you going with it all?

Jenny: Well, it is, it's hard. Sometimes I feel so frustrated with her that I have to . . . put her in her cot and walk out of the room. Then I feel so . . . guilty, I just don't know what to do . . .

GP: When Ivy just keeps crying and crying, what do you make of it? What do you think she's trying to say to you?

Jenny: I feel like she's saying, 'Come on, Mum, make it better. Why can't you figure out what to do here? You're the mum—you're supposed to know what to do.

GP: What's that like for you?

Jenny: I just feel hopeless. I mean, I feel like I'm a total failure as a mum. It makes me think that someone else would do a much better job than me and give Ivy what she really needs.

GP: They're very hard thoughts to be having. How do you think you're feeling generally, in your spirits?

Jenny: I'm okay I think. I have better days and worse days. I've been a bit teary but I think that's just me being tired.

GP: When you say 'worse days', what's a 'worse day' like for you?

Jenny: On a bad day, just getting out of bed is a struggle. I know I have to because Ivy is crying but it just feels all too hard. I have this sense of dread—like I can't face another day with her. Once I get going it's a little easier. It's a bit like I somehow hang on until it's night again and I can go back to bed.

GP: What's a 'better day' like?

Jenny: Usually I have a little more energy and I can get a few things done, maybe a couple of loads of washing and a bit of shopping. I always feel better if I can achieve something.

GP: In a week, what would you guess is your average ratio of better to worse days—say three and four, or two and five?

Jenny: I think about two better and five worse, but it can vary.

GP: And are there things that you can find to cheer you up on a worse day?

Jenny: Um ... well ... not really ... but then my life's not all that interesting at the moment. There's a lot of feeding, nappies, settling over and over. That's just being a mum, I think.

GP: If you're given the opportunity to do something for yourself or something that you've enjoyed in the past, does it feel like you can enjoy it in your usual way?

Jenny: I know Alan thinks I've lost my sense of humour. He doesn't think I laugh anymore. He's probably right. Everything feels really difficult at the moment. It just feels like you have to get through it somehow.

GP: A lot of mums do feel very tired with the broken sleep and night feeding. Tell me about your sleep.

Jenny: I usually fall asleep really easily—I'm just totally finished by the end of the day. Ivy usually wakes me around 1 am for a feed. Then I find it hard to get back to sleep, which is so frustrating because I know she's going to wake me again around five and I know how exhausted I'm going to be the next day.

GP: What do you think keeps you awake?

Jenny: My mind just seems to go round in circles about every little thing. Anything from what I'm going to make for dinner the next day to thinking about finances and how we'll make ends meet . . . now that I'm not working at all. Then I start worrying about Ivy. Sometimes I get back up and check on her just to make sure she's still okay.

GP: Sometimes when we feel low we can get thoughts about not wanting to be here or just wanting things to stop. Have you found yourself having some of these thoughts?

Jenny (crying): There are times when I just think if something could happen that would make me disappear or take me away from all the worry and being so useless it would be better.

GP: That's a very distressing place to get to. Do you find yourself thinking of ways you could end it all or harm yourself?

Jenny: I sometimes imagine myself just driving straight at the end of the road, or running into a tree.

GP: When you get these thoughts, how strongly do you feel you want to act on them?

Jenny: I never get to the point where I'd actually do it. It just comes into my mind for a moment, but then I push it away.

GP: What do you think stops you?

Jenny: I think deep in my heart I know Ivy needs me. Even if I'm not the best mother in the world, I'm the only mother she's got and I couldn't do that to her—just leave her like that without a mum for her whole life. It would be terrible.

GP: Has there ever been a time when you have hurt yourself or tried to end your life?

Jenny: No, never.

GP: Jenny, I also need to check with you—with Ivy crying for hours the way she has been, sometimes you can get urges to be a bit rougher with her than you might normally, maybe out of frustration or anger. Do you find that happening to you?

Jenny: I can't deny that there are times that I do feel totally at my wit's end. I feel like I want to yell at her to get her to be quiet . . . I just get into such a state . . . but somehow I manage to realise I'm about to lose it and I just walk away.

GP: Has there been a time when you didn't catch yourself in time—when you didn't walk away in time?

Jenny: . . . I'm really ashamed to tell you this. I'm ashamed of myself just thinking about it. One night, it was 2 or 3 in the morning and she wasn't settling no matter what I did. I was just so tired . . . so exhausted, and I started getting hysterical—'Just SHUT UP, SHUT UP!' That's what I was saying to my beautiful baby girl. I didn't mean it; I was so tired.

GP: What happened next?

Jenny: Something made me suddenly see what I was doing and gave me enough sense to get out of that room and go get Alan.

He just took one look at me and jumped out of bed and went to Ivy. I cried myself to sleep, hating myself for what had happened. I felt so terrible. After that I made a promise to myself never to let that happen again, so I just walk away when I start to get that feeling. I feel lousy for having to walk away but it's better than getting to that place again.

SOMATIC SYMPTOMS AS A REFLECTION OF PSYCHOLOGICAL STRAIN

PND may be accompanied by or disguised as physical symptoms. Surprisingly, though feeling very real, such symptoms can be of psychological origin. They usually occur as multiple diffuse physical symptoms, including headaches, disturbed sleep, problems with breathing or heart palpitations, and memory and concentration difficulties. Because of their non-specificity and lack of a diagnostic pattern, the sufferer often thinks that doctors will regard such symptoms as trivial and will think she is foolish, so she decides to wait them out. If she does seek help, some health professionals may begin to suspect a psychological origin for these diffuse symptoms that don't resolve and for which there is no obvious physical cause. In other cases, a mother makes multiple visits to the GP for minor health problems in the baby, which can be a sign that she is feeling unwell herself. An empathic and competent health professional will encourage the mother to consider a psychological explanation and offer her a management plan.

DEVELOPING A BALANCED MANAGEMENT PLAN

Factors such as a woman's denial of her difficulties or her translation of them (unconsciously) into physical symptoms makes the health practitioner's diagnostic and formulating tasks more difficult, but it is not beyond a skilled clinician. The greater difficulty is having the mother concede or accept the diagnosis and its implications.

Skilled practitioners should be able to diagnose PND, identify a subtype for the particular mood disorder and weigh the potential causes. In addition, they should explore the woman's coping skills, risk factors, life story and views on mental problems, and respect her beliefs about medication and non-medication therapies for psychological problems. They should also seek her permission to interview a close relative to obtain further information. At the end of that process, they should have a working diagnosis and some hypotheses about causes and contributions (the formulation, see the box above) and a sense of the woman's views (especially about mental health issues).

Once this is completed, it is possible for the health practitioner and the woman in question to design a management plan together. Negotiation is needed. For example, if an antidepressant medication is the best option, at least initially, but the woman refuses to take medication, deciding the best way forward requires skill and subtlety on the part of the health practitioner. Failure to agree on a unified management approach can set in train a cascade of management problems.

Jose's story: finding a way forward

Let's return to Jose (see Chapter 2, page 31), whose distress led to a cry for help from her husband Max.

Clearly, Jose has PND: she has recently had a baby and now appears significantly depressed. It is highly unlikely to be the baby blues, as she has suffered some level of depression for eight years.

Who should Max and Jose consult to formulate what's going on and a way forward? Many mental health professionals do not believe in making a diagnosis, and instead focus more on the patient's life story. Or they concentrate only on a particular aspect—maybe the new baby's disruption collided with Jose's need for order and achievement, or perhaps they consider that Jose's mothering of her newborn has reactivated longstanding conflicts with her own mother. There is a risk of error if the focus is *only* on the life story or *only* on the stressors. The health professional needs to analyse the data to generate a diagnosis, while noting and respecting the patient's narrative and life story.

In managing depression, many health professionals have a single or preferred treatment approach (be it medication, psychotherapy or counselling) and apply it regardless of the patient's actual condition. As our colleague Edward Shorter has observed, 'If all you have is a hammer then everything looks like a nail.' Ideally, your GP should refer you to a practitioner whose therapeutic approach includes many treatment modalities and who knows when a particular treatment type should be the priority. Actually finding such a practitioner can be extremely difficult, however, and often it is facilitated by word of mouth, when a sufferer seeks advice from others who've had a similar problem and found a professional they can recommend.

Now you have read Max's letter about Jose, our chapter covering differing perinatal conditions and the chapter on risk factors. Do you favour a particular diagnosis and formulation, have views about management priorities, thoughts about who should assess Jose (GP, psychiatrist, psychologist, counsellor, mothercraft nurse, alternative practitioner, and so on), and what might be the likely treatment approach?

We hope that what we have outlined has narrowed the diagnostic options. There is no suggestion of a puerperal psychosis—nor of a bipolar disorder, despite her brother having received such a diagnosis. Jose displays the features of a persistent depression that has worsened in recent months (and a family history of mood disorders), with current features of lack of energy, profound insomnia, a despairing non-reactive mood and a hint of suicidal thinking. The most likely diagnosis is melancholic depression.

Now let us take you through the thoughts of the doctor who received this call for help. He judged that a melancholic depression was the probable diagnosis and that Jose would be most likely to benefit from medication. That narrowed the range of people to whom he could refer Jose to health professionals who can prescribe medication—GPs and psychiatrists.

The doctor also noted that Jose sought to deny any problems and viewed mental illness as a stigma. Would referral to a psychiatrist be too threatening to Jose's world view? Referral to a GP colleague would be less stigmatising. While GPs vary in their interest and sophistication in assessing mental health problems, including mood disorders, some have undertaken extra training in the mental health area, and can offer longer consultations for mental health assessments. Jose's doctor elected to discuss the options—GP colleague or psychiatrist—with her. Jose knew her GP socially and said she would prefer to see a psychiatrist.

The psychiatrist confirmed a diagnosis of melancholia and persuaded a reluctant Jose to take an antidepressant, with some psychological strategies planned to accompany this as soon as her mood showed improvement. Two weeks later, Jose's depression had lifted almost completely and she pressed the psychiatrist to cease the medication. The psychiatrist knew the value of the medication, not only in lifting Jose's depression but also in preventing a relapse, but she was also aware of Jose's views about stigma. Jose's resolute personality style of seeking to control her own world while 'not under the influence of drugs' was also a factor to consider. They discussed the issues, trying to reconcile their two viewpoints. After a detailed discussion about the pros and cons of taking medication, Jose agreed to take the antidepressant for a year while also engaging in psychological treatment (with the psychiatrist or a psychologist) and, subject to the stressors in her life settling down and her adopting some non-drug strategies (such as yoga, meditation and exercise), that then she would slowly taper off the medication and return for a review some months after ceasing it completely.

SUMMARY
1. The professional chosen for treatment is very important. We detail the skills of professionals from differing disciplines in Chapter 8.
2. A professional skilled in dealing with perinatal conditions should operate to a biopsychosocial framework (see Chapter 2) in deriving a diagnosis and formulation.
3. The professional should outline the treatment modalities they intend to prioritise (or implement sequentially) and encourage discussion, so that the management plan is jointly owned.

4. While there is substantial evidence that various treatments for PND work, this information is derived from groups of subjects rather than individuals. This makes prediction of how well a particular woman will respond to a treatment course problematic. This means that the professional may, at times, have to change or preferably tweak their management plans.

five

Protecting yourself with realistic expectations

The baby had his mother's eyes, his mother's nose, and his mother's mouth. Which left his mother with a pretty blank expression.

Robert Benchley

Producing and raising children ranks as one of the most demanding roles in a woman's life. Women who are newly pregnant or new mothers are enveloped in expectations and either smothered with advice or taken for granted. Unnoticed at best, criticised at worst, they are required to manage quite extraordinary deeds every day.

In addition to all the body changes and pressures associated with pregnancy, social pressures seem to be increasing. Take just one example—the competitive girth game.

PREGNANCY AS A COMPETITIVE SPORT

And you have no choice but to play for nine long months. There are many individual categories: Who Got Pregnant Most Easily; Most Weight Gained; Least Weight Gained; Most Unpleasant Pregnancy Symptoms; Size and Shape of Bump; Best Pregnancy Wardrobe; Sexiest Pregnancy; Least Pregnant-looking Pregnant Woman. And that's before you even give birth.

Pregnant celebrities and the genuflecting glossy gossip media aren't helping. In fact, they seem to have turned pregnancy into an industry as well as a sport . . . Nobody explains this before you get knocked up. Foolishly, you thought pregnancy was about having a baby, not trying to look like a slightly bloated Victoria's Secret model. Now you know . . .

Not only do you have to be sexy when you're pregnant, you also have to be thin. Not your tummy. Well, not entirely. So long as you're thin everywhere else and just look as if you have a small netball stuck under your shirt, that's okay. You must also glow and look yummy. A yummy pre-mummy.

After giving birth to your netball and peeling off your pregnancy Spanx, the real fun begins. It's time to 'bounce back'! This means erasing all physical evidence that you've ever gestated a human being.

If you're famous, be sure to leave hospital in skinny jeans and industrial Spanx with pert boobs and a spray tan. Somewhere along the way, someone has confused giving birth with a holiday on the Gold Coast.

Mia Freedman[1]

THE CHALLENGES OF BECOMING A PARENT

My days were filled with the demands of a toddler and the background drone of a baby who sounded like a day at the Grand Prix.

Sammy

Women's expectations of themselves as mothers can be immense. No fact sheet can cover the uncertainties of a troubled pregnancy or the feelings that can beset a mum when it's rainy, the baby's unsettled and their favourite GP is off for a few months—maybe, ironically, on maternity leave. Women commonly blame themselves for not managing as seamlessly as, it seems to them, other women do. The reality is that other women may be hiding their true feelings just as effectively.

Starting with pregnancy and intensifying when the new baby is brought home, there is a tsunami of changes in the lives of each new mother, her partner and her relatives and friends. Yet there's something of a conspiracy of silence about the massive impact of these changes. Precisely because having a child is so commonplace, myths and expectations cluster unhelpfully around pregnancy, birth and the baby's first year, leaving the new mother and her partner rather stranded. If the new family asks for or needs extra support at this time it can be seen as an admission of failure—though usually more by the mother herself than by others.

Why, at one of the times of greatest vulnerability and huge adjustments mentally and physically, in a lifetime involvement of immense importance for which they have had little or no training, are most pregnant women or newly minted young parents expected to be able to figure things out for themselves? Suddenly they alone are responsible for round-the-clock care of a young person who is totally dependent on them, with no break in sight for years! And why is it so rarely acknowledged that it is the rule, not the exception, for mothers and fathers in this situation to occasionally lose their footing, get dumped by a wave and struggle to stay afloat? A lifesaver would be on call in a corresponding situation.

The difficulties for dads

The new father can be overlooked in the hubbub surrounding the pregnancy and birth. He's had to make some massive changes to his life, too. If he can spend real time caring for the baby, not just babysitting, it can transform this feeding/eating/crying/excreting tot into an individual the new dad begins to read.

Frank weighs in with some pragmatic male observations about his first attempts to take some of the load from his frazzled wife. He felt lost and all thumbs with their newborn—before he adjusted and started to provide practical help. His wife's anxiety meant that she had become obsessively involved with every detail of the baby's care, and the more this happened, the less room there was for anyone else to care for the baby in exactly the way she felt was essential. Frank negotiated with her and took over parts of the routine, which allowed him to carve out a trusted space for his relationship with the baby, and provide support for her:

I don't mind telling you that I felt like a teat on a bull for a while there. I was learning to manage our little fellow just like my wife was but she was too worried about him to let me do much. He cried a lot when we got him home and she was getting more and more tired and cranky so I said, 'Look, love, let's work out some times when you're okay to leave me with the baby.'

So it got that I'd look after him while she had a shower, and then after work I'd take him for a spin around the block while she put dinner on or, better still, I'd pick up some takeaway food at the same time. He was good for me. We got on real well. Next my wife and I agreed that on Saturday and Sunday I'd get him out of the house as soon as she'd finished his 6 am feed and so she was able to hit the sack again for two hours. I got to know all the shift workers in the neighbourhood!

And she didn't get shirty then when I'd cut loose and go to the footy with mates.

Greater interaction between father and baby can make the intense first few months more rewarding for the new father and also foster his relationship with his partner. His active support reduces the fuel for resentment and blame that can flare in tired new parents when, for example, the baby starts up just as they're about to have dinner.

It's normal to voice some frustrations

Sometimes new parents themselves are caught up in the need to preserve the rosy vision. It seems so negative to grizzle about the occasional (sometimes frequent) downsides of this novel situation—parenthood. Yet it can be so helpful for a new mother and her spouse to talk about and normalise the difficulties and how they're feeling about them. It's not negative to be frank about the hardships. It doesn't detract from the wonder and fascination of the baby. In fact, being realistic brings perspective, stamina and balance, and an opportunity for both parents to pinpoint the more difficult times and negotiate possible solutions.

While the majority of mothers and their partners adjust well to pregnancy and parenting, at least a third of mothers find the adjustment disabling and more than merely challenging. This is not only with their first child; it can happen with subsequent pregnancies and toddlers. Women have to form their identity as a mother—even those who were the mainstay for their smaller sisters and brothers in earlier years, even those who have dealt with babies and children extensively as part of their profession. Many are surprised to find that past experience counts for little at 2 am when, near dead with exhaustion, they are faced with their own baby who just won't settle.

Resentment, love, ambivalence, all at once

I must smile when I go to pick her up—she hasn't woken on purpose just to interrupt what I'm doing.

Taylor

The elephant in the room is that both the mother and her partner are likely to have occasional feelings of resentment towards the baby. It's hard not to: you're so tired, the baby seems so demanding. You may feel ambivalence during this testing time (remember when you could simply walk out the door when you felt like it?) but it's possible, and necessary, to hold two contradictory views at the same time: the baby is the sun in your universe but now, earth-like, you're in a fixed orbit for a while!

You don't need to be perfect parents

Home at last. But newly minted parents can find themselves faced with a hurdle—one of their own making. Parents want to give their baby a psychologically perfect start in life. At the same time they have become hyper-aware of every nuance of child raising, via the flood of readily available information. This may lead them to set unrealistic goals. For instance, they vow they will never express negative emotion around their baby, or feel they must be constantly attentive, present and engaged with their child. The late Dr Donald Winnicott, a paediatrician and psychoanalyst, was one of the first to research the effects of parenting on infants, and contended that parents did not need to be perfectly attuned, just 'good enough' to protect the baby from too often experiencing extremes of discomfort and distress, either emotional or physical. The 'good enough parent' is not a 'second-best' parent—they are likely to be more realistic, pragmatic and relaxed.

The toughest job in the world?

A baby: the gift that keeps on taking . . .

Anon.

Society idealises mothers. We are bombarded with prettified images and success stories via magazine articles, television and film and advertisements, but for real parents society is fractured, busy and impersonal. It can provide a somewhat noxious setting for a young family. The perplexing harsh reality for mothers is that there is pervasive, albeit unconscious, discrimination. This discrimination is too subtle to identify and fight, and it comes at a time when its victim has little energy, capacity, confidence or influence to demand redress. Better subsidised child care, more affordable kindergartens, more sympathetic work patterns, family-friendly public spaces, more readily available public transport and improved links to community support would all help.

Consider the following job parameters crafted by Donna.

WANTED—CANDIDATES FOR MOTHERHOOD

Imagine being given the most important job in the world (to you anyway). This job is not explained in any detail but will change your life forever. You can't relinquish this job once you have agreed to take it on. You may begin it feeling sick, sore and exhausted. You're not sure about what you're supposed to do or when—indeed, it seems you should 'know' instinctively. There is no boss or feedback—and if you ask for advice it's firmly given and usually in conflict with what others have told you!

You will be expected to carry out this job mostly in isolation, behind closed doors, using your own resourcefulness. The working conditions are pretty tough: you're 'on' 24/7, all of every day for the foreseeable future, without financial reward, certainly no salary . . . and for at least 18 years.

It is, however, a vital job with very important downstream consequences. There is a critical audience (at least you may think so, and you may be right) whom you must present with results—and results that accord with their expectations.

When you have accepted the job you may find that the baby you've been given doesn't respond to your dedicated project management and has been issued with neither a 'how to' manual nor a gauge in its forehead to help you judge whether it's getting enough sustenance. You can't turn it off either.

Pregnancy and motherhood are certainly a big ask and a huge financial investment, yet millions of women consider this their right and privilege. It's the most popular and sought-after job in the world. Expertise as a parent supposedly arrives with the baby, but motherhood is as much an art as a science. There is too much time given, perhaps, to the birth, and not enough to shaping the skills that are called on from day one of motherhood.

MOTHERS NEGLECTING THEMSELVES

Mothers probably take more care of their washing machines, not overloading them, letting them cool down, not putting too much washing powder in . . . it's not a great example, but you know what I mean. You're not a machine. Just try to spot the wear and tear before you rust out!

Cassie

Women who are pregnant, have just given birth or are in the first few years of raising young children are often too distracted or busy to look after themselves. Studies find that mothers know the importance of taking care of their own emotional and physical needs, and that an unhealthy mother is ultimately a less effective mother. Conflicting with this belief, though, is the conviction that selflessness is synonymous with good parenting.[2] Organising time and routines to lighten the extra physical and psychological demands can be difficult, reflecting the dictates of any other children, varying levels of support from partners or coping without a partner, and unavailable (or too expensive) support.

Additionally, mothers are unhelpfully bombarded with images of 'yummy mummies' who have miraculously returned to their svelte selves two weeks after giving birth—an ideal that is disconcerting at best. In the pursuit of these 'ideals', some women take themselves beyond the boundaries of good health.

There are many warnings and much stern advice out there but actually finding support, understanding and a sympathetic ear may be harder. Of course we all have bad days. But when, during the perinatal time, does a bad day become a succession of bad days; become a bigger problem—but still manageable; become a problem that *could* be fixed and distress eased; become a problem that *needs* to be fixed; become a problem that *has* to be fixed?

The central paradox

Here's a paradox. Why is it that many women who find pregnancy or early motherhood daunting don't seek help and refuse it if it is offered? These women often adopt a mask and stay behind it, hoping their 'show face' will protect them from both the real and imaginary consequences of opening up about their distress. Some women's masks are so firmly in place they fool even themselves.

THE MASK OF MOTHERHOOD

A pregnant woman or a mother during the first year after birth often:

- *Does* know that she is having difficulties that are eroding her satisfaction with becoming/being a mother.
- *Doesn't* recognise that such difficulties are more often the rule than the exception, blames herself, keeps quiet and struggles on.

Women who find pregnancy or motherhood difficult can become shy, reclusive and very private. Because of the motherhood myths, they do not feel licensed to admit to doubts and problems—even to themselves. Understandably, women are extremely vulnerable at this time and many fear that their difficulties with parenting will be exposed for all to see—and also seen as abnormal.

Reasons women don't seek help

Women often have trouble setting boundaries—staking out space for themselves. As one said:

My husband just goes and has a shower. Why can't I do the same? What I do instead, I either ask him to look after the baby while blaming him for not 'mindreading' (I'm thinking I shouldn't have to ask for help, he should be able to see it's needed) or I tie myself in knots setting up a time to shower while the baby is asleep. Why don't I just tell him and then do it? I think I get into these situations because I feel a bit worn down and sorry for myself.

As well as the muddle that comes from being chronically tired, other reasons for not asking for help include fears about appearing incapable, losing control of a situation when others provide counterintuitive advice, the risk of feeling rejected if the request is met with a 'no' or being seen as a burden if there is a 'yes'. That's a lot of energy knotted up that could be better used for the baby. One mother observed, 'We fear putting people out but in reality people love to be needed, especially if we tell them the specific help they can provide.'

The above observations give rise to two dilemmas. First, how can we convince women that there is help available and that, in accessing it, they are not on some slippery slope that automatically leads to intrusive exposure to well-meaning 'authorities'? (If they can make use of assistance before they become too worn down, it empowers them to return to their all-absorbing passion—mothering their baby and any other children.) Secondly, how can those who care extend a helping hand if a woman having difficulties can't trust herself or them enough to reach out and grasp it?

PERINATAL MOOD PROBLEMS RESPOND VERY WELL TO HELP

Our approach is direct. This book includes some disturbing details of perinatal depression but, by including such accounts, we aim to set out some of the clinical reasoning adopted by skilled health professionals whom readers might approach for advice. The great majority of perinatal mood problems dissipate spontaneously or, with appropriate management, more rapidly than if left untreated. There is always hope. We have presented a frank examination of the clinical features of mood disorders, risk factors and predictors of good outcomes. Every story in this book endorses the fact that it was when women or their partners first sought and accepted help that they gained access to a wealth of support that enabled them to regain their own equilibrium and allowed them to parent better.

ACCEPT HELP AND ALLOW YOURSELF TO BE 'GOOD ENOUGH'

Resist the 'shoulds' of motherhood by considering a broader set of counterviews:

1. Don't say, 'I can manage, thanks'

Where's the rule that says a new mother has to do it all herself? Please ask for and accept help. What have other new mothers found to be of benefit? Judge how and when others can lend a hand. Help those who want to assist by defining how they can best fit in, what they can do and when.

When a friend asks 'Is there anything I can do to help?' say, 'Yes—could you help with XX chores, or hold the baby while I have a shower?'

2. Don't promise yourself not to cut corners

Don't prioritise being perfect above being good enough. Ditch the Superwoman cape. Beware the scourge of feeding your friends homemade cake in your spotless house. Anyone on your side won't be running a finger over the windowsills to check for dust. Who does that anyway, and if they do, do you really want them for a friend or think you should listen to them?

3. Don't say, 'I'll attend to my own health . . . later'
Before you can supply the needs of another, especially a baby, you need to make sure your own battery is full. *Never* miss the opportunity for a sleep, any amount. Sleep should come first, second and third. Then try to add in some exercise. And think how you can best nourish your body. You're still recuperating from a Very Big Event (remember, the birth?). Birth, breastfeeding, the resetting of hormones and involuntary sleep deprivation all merit recovery time.

4. Don't tell yourself that motherhood is instinctive or that there *is* a right way
It can't be both and in fact it's neither. Instinct is not commonplace but your intuition *is* in there. After being all thumbs for a while, you'll gradually recognise your little one's routines and what seems to work. Think about the fact that childcare nurses require years of training to become competent in the job of looking after babies! Getting into as much of a pattern as possible means that at least you know what *you're* doing!

5. Don't tell yourself it's wrong to run off to doctors
With a bit of luck, your understanding and available GP (if they're not, find another), will become your new best friend. Develop a trusting relationship—drop the mask and be honest. Visit as often as you need for the baby but also tell the doctor how *you* are. If you are developing a slew of physical symptoms—tiredness, headaches, a churning stomach—give some thought to whether you're under too much pressure and whether such symptoms reflect your psychological rather than your physical state.

6. Don't say, 'Making time for myself is selfish'
Arrange some time for yourself without the baby and/or other children. Use it to chill out, recharge your battery and confirm

that you (and your partner) are still there. And exercise (with and without baby, preferably every day) is an essential, not a luxury. You'll be all the better as a mother as you come back through the front door.

7. Don't tell yourself, 'The birth must be "natural" ' or 'Breastfeeding comes naturally'

'Instinctive' and 'natural' are words much bandied about during pregnancy and the baby's first year. Beware: they're spring-loaded and can hurt you. Birth is a big undertaking and it is an exceptional birth that doesn't require *some* medical intervention. Yet some mothers ruminate and rehash the birth of their baby when it didn't go according to plan. If you're one of these mums, see if you can sort out why you're upset and then move on—or talk it through with someone who can help. Try not to invest energy in upset or regrets—you need that energy for all the other things you're doing.

The same goes for breastfeeding. Unless you're taking a particular medication that prevents you from breastfeeding, persist with it if possible, and speak to a breastfeeding helpline or get a nurse to visit you at home if it's not working out. Congratulate yourself if it does. Remind yourself, however, breastfeeding isn't for everyone and the baby will be *fine* if you decide to bottle-feed. There are some quasi-religious beliefs surrounding birth and breastfeeding that breed strong attitudes and loads of judgement and advice that can sap rather than support you. Be as pragmatic as possible.

8. Don't promise yourself, 'I will always be patient and unflustered'

You may feel guilty no matter what you do—motherhood can do that to a woman—so try not to obsess about any perceived mistake. Sometimes, too, a part of you can make you uncomfortably aware of and vulnerable to others' opinions. Fix any slip-up or forget it, but *move on*. There are going to be days when you think you're a hopeless mother and that every other mother is totally in command. You're not. And they aren't.

9. Don't think, 'I should behave impeccably or the baby's psyche will be affected'

You're the *only* mother your baby knows or wants. You have their best interests at heart and know them better than anyone in the world. A mother can only ever be 'good enough'. And that is good enough. You can't damage your baby with momentary lapses of attentiveness or composure. If you feel unsure, seek and accept help: it can provide invaluable perspective and self-management skills that will be yours for life.

10. Don't think you shouldn't reach out

There is a community out there with resources, tips and strategies at its fingertips: your local mothers' group. Share their expertise: they are new mums just like you. Often you can meet a couple of other mums from the group separately, allowing friendships and support to grow.

Use your community centre or the last healthcare worker you liked to track down a mothers' group—or perhaps the mums you were in hospital with will know of one. Ensure that it is a supportive, not a competitive group. Go twice and then, if that mothers' group still looks bulletproof, find another group that's more you. (Avoid mothers' groups where they seem to vie with each other for best baby, quickest bounce-back after birth and longest sleep through the night.)

If you've been feeling pretty down, you may be referred to a mothers' group where the mums are feeling the same way. These women can become the most valuable friends you'll ever make.

six

Learning to live in motherland

Immediately following birth, every new mother drags herself from her bed and awkwardly pulls herself up on the pedestal provided for her. Some adjust easily to the saintly image. Some can't stand the heights and jump off, never to be seen again. But most mothers just try to figure out what they're supposed to do—and how they can do it in public.

Erma Bombeck[1]

A woman embarking on pregnancy, birth and motherhood will experience mixed emotions. The romanticised shiny mum-to-be 'eating for two', the magazine depiction of celebrities displaying their elegant baby bump, the new mums plus latest model pram pursuing their post-birth bounce-back all capture an idealised fantasy. While for most parents it is a time of joy, there has to be space and permission to acknowledge and validate some of the knocks along the way.

THE AMBIVALENCE OF MOTHERHOOD
One GP, a mum herself, observed:

There can be an underlying confusion and ambivalence that accompanies the conflicting experience of 'my baby is miraculous and wondrous' and 'I am terrified, bewildered and depleted'. The idea that these two are not mutually exclusive truths often offers relief and validation to parents who feel that, if they subscribe to the latter set of thoughts, they are denouncing the first.[2]

Mei Lin was already aware of the tension between how she actually felt and how others thought she should feel. She knew that if her ambivalence became more pronounced, she would have to justify her feelings . . . or disguise them:

> *How to convey the negative thoughts that crowd your brain when you discover for the first time: 'I'm pregnant!'*
>
> *You're supposed to be ecstatic. Anything less is a betrayal to all those people who can't have children or try for years on IVF.*
>
> *But what if you're less than ecstatic?*
>
> *What if you immediately think: 'I'm not ready for this. It was a mistake. I haven't got my own act together yet. Is my relationship strong enough to cope with this? How will I give birth? What if something is wrong with the baby?'*

DEPRESSION DURING PREGNANCY

Depression was thought to be uncommon during pregnancy, until the findings from the 2001 Avon study.[3] This longitudinal (long-term) study assessed women from pregnancy, and the women and their offspring for more than 20 years. Surprisingly, women's rates of 'probable' depression were higher during pregnancy than after the birth. Further studies have also found high rates of distress or depression-like symptoms during pregnancy.

While undoubtedly some pregnant women *are* depressed, a number of the symptoms overlap with aspects of the pregnancy itself—for example, low energy, poor sleep, weight change and heightened emotionality.[4] Women sleep poorly during pregnancy, not necessarily because they're depressed but simply because they're pregnant,[5] and their poor sleep can lead to some depression-like symptoms or increased levels of body chemicals that can cause those symptoms. So when symptoms arise in pregnancy, you and your doctor should consider whether the cause is depression, the pregnancy itself and/or disturbances in sleep and sleep quality.

Knowing is not the same as feeling

Tanya was well prepared and realistic about what to expect during her first months with her new baby. Being prepared intellectually, though very useful in and of itself, didn't equate to being prepared for the range of emotions that were brought into play after the birth. Tanya and her husband were very happy about their little one but even so there were days when she couldn't help thinking, 'What have we done?' Some days she found herself grieving—mourning the loss of her old life, youthful figure, independence, unbroken sleep, social life, semi-disposable income and wonderful job. Other days, she wouldn't have had it any other way:

Throughout my pregnancy, I prepared thoroughly. I read and read, I attended antenatal classes, and my husband and I did a marriage course to work on things like communication and conflict resolution. As well as talking to friends about what the initial months were like, I even arranged for us to have coffee with a couple who had experienced severe postnatal depression. I blogged about how I was feeling physically and mentally. I purchased a smartphone because you could operate it one-handed and use its social media capabilities to get support or find company during lonely night feeds.

Nine months passed and delivery day came. After six hours of uncomplicated labour we got to meet our little girl and our family expanded to three. From the beginning, it wasn't as bad as I'd feared. I discovered I had a fairly happy baby who fed well, slept well and only cried for good reason.

Nevertheless, further down the track, when most of the attention, interest and concern had died down, I found myself struggling. Some days were relaxed, other days I felt trapped but couldn't pinpoint what was wrong. Some days I embraced motherhood, other days I wondered if I had done the right thing in quitting work and felt irrationally compelled to ring my boss to beg for my job back. Some days my husband and I were united, working shoulder to shoulder as Team Awesome Parents, other days we sniped at each other and argued about the right way to do things. Above all, I wondered who—or what—I was now. A milk factory? A housewife? A burden on society?

Unlike some women, motherhood did not come naturally to me. Aside from clothing, feeding, changing and bathing my baby, I did not quite know what to 'do' with her. I was a classic introvert who was used to spending my days alone in my office, so being around someone else all the time was really confronting. I had friends with kids, but I didn't really understand the full nature of what family life was like. The mothers I knew seemed to disappear off the face of the earth after giving birth, and when they resurfaced months—or even years—later I'd ask how things were going and they would reply in vague platitudes that offered no insight into their experiences.

Furthermore, I found the options available in Mummyland were most unsatisfactory. Which altar would I choose? Would I sacrifice myself on the altar of family, or continue in the workplace and sacrifice our family time on the altar of career? There seemed to be no middle way.

ADAPTING AND ATTUNING

Feedback: When the baby doesn't appreciate the strained carrots.

Anon.

Motherhood can be like moving permanently to a new and challenging country. According to Bethany in her piece, 'Negotiating Motherland', you may have visited Motherland on a tourist visa (as an aunt or godparent) but that's very different from the experience of actually living there. That requires a whole different level of acclimatisation:

Becoming a mother for the first time reminds me of going to live in India. There is jet lag, which in Motherland lasts for approximately 23 years. You don't speak the local language. You don't understand the transport system. Time has changed: suddenly the ten things you could get done in a day may, possibly, be accomplished in a month. There is culture shock, which in itself is a shock because, first of all, you are a woman and isn't this what women do? And you have read all the guide books, spoken to experienced travellers, seen snapshots, documentaries, home movies, and perhaps even been on the Contiki tour of 'Aunt' and 'Godparent'.

But visiting India is not like living in India. Motherland can't be simulated, and going to live there for the first time is daunting. And beginning motherhood with a mood disorder is like going to live in India and simultaneously developing malaria—you may be extremely happy to be there but you don't really feel like unpacking your suitcase and tucking into some local cuisine!

My first pregnancy ended in a miscarriage. My body went from being a cradle of hope and excitement to a grave. My flight to Motherland had been cancelled while I was sitting on the plane. I soon found myself in the chaos of being somewhere but not having any idea where. I went to work and social events as usual but always felt a profound sense of incompetence. I perceived disapproval in the slightest eyebrow-raise or heavy exhale. I'd come home and cry or yell or artfully do both at the same time. It wasn't until over a year later that I visited a counsellor to settle myself.

I conceived a second time. As the pregnancy continued, despite relentless morning sickness with a chaser of heartburn, I felt well. And after the birth things continued relatively well. I do remember the claustrophobic realisation, 'Oh my goodness, this person literally needs me every three to four hours, 24 hours a day,' and the baffling bombardment of conflicting advice on what seemed like every decision I had to make. But this culture shock was far outweighed by feelings of love and happiness at having my newborn son in my life. I liked being here.

Then, when my son was around eight months, I happily became pregnant for the third time. With this pregnancy, however, the morning sickness came with mood swings, anxiety, irritability and inability to make decisions. It's not that my love had turned off, nor that I didn't want to be a mother anymore, but my confidence in negotiating the terrain had taken a backslide.

To accommodate the coming baby we bought a house and moved closer to family. Packing the last of our things appeared to be a simply impossible undertaking. I felt I had to do something to shore myself up to manage this next leg of the journey. I sought and received counselling from our local public hospital and my due date became a finishing line, providing a definite and approaching end.

Since my daughter's birth, my moods have slowly improved. How do I account for this? Perhaps I have acclimatised, becoming more adept at living in Motherland. The landscape itself has become less treacherous and I'm more sure-footed because of increased sleep, some time to myself, reduced demand for breastfeeding, fewer fluctuating hormones.

But I like to think that, through continuing to see a counsellor and personal quiet times with my version of God, I have also learned some ways of being that have helped me find resources in myself I never knew were there.

Establishing sleeping and eating patterns

People who say they sleep like a baby usually don't have one.

Leo J. Burke

At the end of a long pregnancy, especially those last tiring weeks when the bump decides to do a bit of exercise the moment you lie down to rest—not to mention what, if you have one, your toddler might be up to—you need every last bit of energy to actually produce the baby. As they say, it's fun getting it in there but hard work getting it out. Anyway, you're home with the new baby and pretty pleased with how you're going. Sure, you're a bit knocked about, but you're proud to be still standing. Our apologies here to those mums who've had a really rough time of it—you're probably already bushwhacked.

What every mum needs now is sleep. Hmmm. Babies vary a lot in their sleep requirements—the average is 16 hours in every 24, but who's ever had the 'average' baby? The actual range lies between eight and 22 hours a day. The babies who sleep for 20 hours a day and only wake for a feed have all gone home with other people—leaving you with yours.

Initially, experts say, until your milk supply is established, babies prefer to feed at night. Many are fairly insatiable when their mother's milk first comes in (around two and a half days). This usually happens about 12 hours after you begin to feel changes in your breasts. And there are some cues to help you determine how well the baby latches onto the breast. During a feed, a few short, rapid sucks should be followed by slower, deeper sucks, with occasional pauses before the sucking starts again without your intervention. A baby who goes to sleep is probably not latched on.

A feeding baby has his/her head tipped back and chin touching your breast with the nose free to enable easy breathing. Some of your areola should still be visible, with more above your baby's top lip than below the bottom lip. It might be useful to identify only a couple of sources of information you trust rather than try to navigate the ocean of other advice.[6]

After a few days, babies start to sleep more during the night—in theory, anyway! Rosemary, now a grandmother, recounts her experience with her toddler (currently the energetic director of an advertising firm), who seemingly never slept:

> We safety-proofed Luke's room and the house to the nth degree because he was awake so much longer than we could be. For the first 18 months we thought we could outstay him. We did relays over the nights. He was cheerful, never cried much; he just wanted to be up and at it. When he was older, one or the other of us would often be found halfway through the fifth story book fast asleep on his bed while he contentedly played nearby.
>
> One night—he must have been about 2 years old—he came in, quite politely, to wake us. It was 3 am. He had been exploring the drawers in his room and had managed to don quite a tasteful selection of clothes, including a beach hat, but he indicated that he needed help to put on some gloves he had found. I must admit to roaring at him, 'Go back to bed. Daddy and I just have to SLEEP!'
>
> He never seemed disturbed by our occasional wild-eyed exhaustion, and we're still close. He and his wife now have their own little one. He's dotty about the baby but, he says, 'She never sleeps!'

It is paramount to normalise sleep as much as possible during the perinatal period. We have innate systems that regulate our sleep–wake cycle and our moods throughout the day. These are typically disrupted by shift work and, of course, during the perinatal period. Such disruptions can trigger, worsen and prolong mood states. One study reported that sleeping less than four hours at night and one hour during the day increases vulnerability to depression at three months after the birth.[7] Other research shows that infant sleep problems that persist until the age of 6–12 months are strongly linked to maternal depression, and that strategies that improve infant sleep relieve depression in mothers.

In short, seeking help to improve problematic sleep patterns in your new baby is a practical investment in your own mental health.[8] When mothers and fathers are taught strategies to improve sleep in their infant, maternal stress, anxiety and/or depression levels really improve in response.

Colic . . . and advice about advice

Everyone had answers but me. Shopkeepers, acquaintances, neighbours, parenting books, strangers in the street. Anyone who had been a mother had insider wisdom to pass on. Controlled crying? Attachment parenting? Colic remedies? Solutions poured in and overflowed onto my sterile confusion.

Eliza

There is a 'crying curve', a graph that shows how much the average baby cries. During the early months of the infant's life, crying often increases at around 2–3 weeks, peaks at 6–8 weeks and hits its lowest level around 4 months. By the age of 6 months, the baby may still cry for two hours a day. The average infant cries for between one and five hours of every 24. Babies tend to cry in the late afternoon and early evening—just when you may be feeling a little ropy yourself. Colic is the term used for when a clearly thriving baby has longer than typical periods of unsoothable crying. Colic is *not* an indicator that anything is wrong with your parenting.

One mother observed that crying was a problem every evening in the early months of her daughter's life. At about 6 pm the screams would start. Nothing would pacify her until she finally fell asleep around 11 pm. Another mum, Rosa, wrote:

And still the baby screams. He screams all day. Nights are a little better. I guess he is so exhausted by then he just has to sleep. I make a discovery. The sound of the hairdryer silences him for brief periods of time. I don't know if he is soothed or terrified by it, but it works—for a while. Then one day the hairdryer breaks down and I cry again.

In her book *A Life's Work*, renowned novelist Rachel Cusk says she once fed her baby for nearly two hours. 'That should do it,' she thinks. Yet five minutes later the baby is crying again. As she stares into 'the insatiable red cave' of her daughter's mouth, she tries to unravel the tangle of crying and feeding in which they have become knotted. She reasons that feeding in response to her baby's cries has reached its logical limit.

She pauses:

I try to see things from her point of view. Every time she cries my breasts appear like prison warders investigating a disturbance, two dumb, moonfaced henchmen closing in on her, silencing her, administering opiates. She could be crying because she's tired, or in pain; she could be crying in the attempt to express herself; she could be crying, God knows, with surfeit, crying in order to relocate the silence of satisfaction, of content. I begin to suspect that I have presided over some kind of bureaucratic madness, wherein feeding has become the penalty for crying and hence creates more *crying.*[9]

Everyone has a theory on how to soothe crying babies and how to relieve colic. After checking the baby is getting enough milk, you could investigate the other possible causes and strategies for an apparently colicky baby: such as hunger, cold, tiredness, heat, or a full nappy change, although even a well-fed, clean, well-wrapped and well-cared-for baby can cry. For more on the causes of colic and how to deal with it, try the book *Baby on Board* by Dr Howard Chilton.[10]

ASK YOURSELF: 'HOW AM I GOING?'

The counsellor said to me, 'Some kind of adjustment to parenthood is normal, but it's about teasing out what's normal and what's illness-based.'

Emily

Throughout this book we extend an appeal to mothers and mothers-to-be. Pregnancy and motherhood initiate waves that can build to increasing turbulence. Every woman has *some* difficulty learning how to cope and adapt, and even knowing whether the way they are functioning is normal ('typical' is perhaps the better word). There is no clear boundary. If, however, the stress keeps building, if your confidence or sanity is threatened, if you feel dispirited much of the time and certainly if your world has become a dark place, then we encourage you to seek professional assessment to clarify what's happening.

If you decide to seek support, the first person you see may not turn out to be the person best suited to help you. Don't be discouraged by this. It is imperative that you feel comfortable, and finding the GP, counsellor or psychologist who 'gets you' may take a couple of goes. You could view it as a sort of job interview—you may need to interview a few candidates before you find out who is the best fit for you.

SOME REASSURANCE—AND A MESSAGE

Much of the stress and tension around a new baby is natural adjustment to a massive change; it settles with time. Difficulties in motherhood can most often be sorted out and assisted without the stigma of turning them into an illness. There is help from your GP, community nurse, community baby care centre and family. When stress and tension become severe, persistent and disabling, however, professional assessment will provide relief and stronger support.

The message in this book—and a constant plea from our essayists—is that enlisting extra support is *not* an admission of failure. It will strengthen you as a mother and, by extension, the whole family. It will increase your ability to become the parent you hoped to be.

seven

Do you need help?

Call your sorrow a disease or don't. Take medications or don't. See a therapist or don't. But whatever you do, when life drives you to your knees, which it is bound to do, which maybe it is meant to do, don't settle for being sick in the brain.

Gary Greenberg[1]

While perinatal mood disorders are common, around 50 per cent of women with these conditions go undiagnosed and do not receive treatment. Like any disease, mood disorders can become more severe and harder to treat the longer they are left untreated, and their collateral damage accrues—to the mother, her relationships (especially the bond with her baby and with her partner) and her capacity to function. Denial is the enemy of recovery.

HOW CAN YOU TELL IF YOU'RE DEPRESSED?
While access to diagnosis and treatment is more readily available now, this poignant essay illustrates that many still experience considerable problems. Susannah recently suffered very significant depression that went undiagnosed. It eventually dissipated without treatment but, like depression in general and untreated depression in particular, it can leave a different and scarred individual in its wake.

Susannah observed that when things go wrong it is usually possible to identify points along the way at which someone could have intervened. She knew that at times she 'dropped the mask and tentatively tried to get help from people who were trained, paid and employed to provide it'. They failed to see her suffering or chose not to—perhaps reflecting their own attitude towards mental illness. Susannah records:

It began in hospital, where my baby and I fell through the cracks of a cohesive care plan, handballed from one blasé agency nurse to the next. Later there was the maternal health nurse, who told me at three weeks that the baby had lost weight. She looked at me closely and asked how I was coping. When I hesitantly opened my mouth to explain, she noted a time in her book for me to see her the next day. When I arrived, feeling that at last someone would listen to me, she was not there. Instead, another nurse brusquely told me that I would just have to feed him more often than three-hourly. There was no follow-up.

At a six-week check with the obstetrician I voiced my feelings of failure and shame. He looked at a spot over my head and told me that it wasn't my fault that I'd finished up with an emergency caesarean. I took my son to his routine visit to the paediatrician and asked if babies were affected when their mothers couldn't really love them. He told me that it sometimes took a while for the mother–baby bond to develop.

My first months of motherhood were fraught with corrosive anxiety and an aching, inexplicable sadness from which there was no respite. The people around me at that time were either oblivious to my sense of hopelessness or powerless to help me. Looking back, I can see that their unresponsiveness was at least partly due to my determination to keep these feelings to myself. I needed to be perceived as a good mother, even though I felt that I was dying inside.

On paper, I presented as a clever, capable adult woman. I wonder if this competence and maturity left me more vulnerable, more likely to be beset by events and feelings over which I had no control, pressured by other people's expectations of me and my own expectations of myself. I know that once my baby was born, I was in an unfamiliar place. My desire for order and tendency towards perfectionism, rather than helping me swim against the tide, sucked me into a whirlpool. My skills of close reading, of analysis and deconstruction, were of no use to me here. I had some insight; I could perceive and understand some aspects of my situation, but was powerless to address it. This was uncharted country: all the looked-for signposts were missing.

A friend once described her depression to me as 'like living with gloves on'. Everything is dulled, muted and blunted. I now know that it is possible to progress through the events of the day without fully engaging with them, to hear news—shocking, joyful or tragic—and struggle to feel anything at all, much less frame a response that is even minimally adequate. It is possible to feed and hold a baby but feel that an impermeable film separates you from him: that it is not really your skin making contact with his. For months I was able to get dressed, answer questions and prepare meals while cocooned in misery and aloneness. Some detached part of me hovered above this automated self, observing, aware, dispassionate and entirely disconnected. My real brain processed information in an isolated bubble while my stiffly smiling puppet-self thought unfamiliar thoughts, inhabited my house, slept in my bed and slowly, effortfully, did most of the things expected of me.

Over time, I emerged from the black fog surrounding me. Sensation gradually began to return to my numbed self. I remember a day when I felt the sun warm on my back as I pushed the pram down the street. I remember the first time I was able to laugh, genuinely and responsively when my son laughed in his bath. I remember being relieved that at the five-month milestone I could prepare vegetable mush and spoon it into his eagerly open mouth. It seemed somehow a positive step away from my abject breastfeeding failure. I remember looking down into my son's smiling eyes and being swamped by love. But it took months.

Postnatal depression was briefly discussed in our antenatal classes. Sitting in a circle, hands folded across our swollen bellies, we were advised to seek help immediately. The premise was that informed, sensitive and compassionate help is readily available. My own experience proves that frequently it is not. My son and I were dismally let down by a whole cohort of people who could and should have responded to us effectively. These included family members and to some extent my partner, although I believe that his mental state became affected by mine. And I think a proportion of mainstream health professionals—as opposed to mental health professionals—do not always recognise altered mind states. Rhetoric and policy are not necessarily mirrored by appropriate action.

I know that I am only one of many women who dwell in a silent community of grief. Our loss is rarely acknowledged. We grieve always for the time that we did not fully have with our babies. Our experience of motherhood encompasses a crippling sense of panic and profound despair.

WHY NEW MOTHERS DON'T RECOGNISE THEIR OWN DEPRESSION

- They have some good days.
- They have a logical reason for being so tired.
- They don't know that depression can also manifest as physical symptoms, overwhelming anxiety or even numbness and lack of feeling, and even if they've previously suffered from depression, their symptoms can differ from episode to episode.
- Because of the joyless dirge in their head (or from their own, maybe depressed mother), 'It's just how motherhood feels.'
- They know that *something's* wrong but they're not sure what it is or what to do about it. Depression itself can erode the ability to communicate and make decisions.
- They don't want to add the stigma of mental illness to feeling like a failure as a mum.

Ellie observed that recognising she had a mood disorder was her first hurdle:

I had a complete lack of understanding of how depression actually manifested itself. People with depression, I naively considered, were melancholy and frequently in torrents of tears. I took months to consider postnatal depression as a possibility. I was not oppressed by a frequent tear-inducing sadness—rather, a gradual decline in the ability to enjoy life. Dissatisfaction pervaded me. I was restless, desperately searching for meaning or purpose and discontented with what I had. Everything and everybody disappointed me—my family, my marriage, my work. I was drowning in the monotony of housework and the all-consuming demands of parenting two children under two. Each day left me more despondent, more restless, than the day before.

Symptoms different from previous episodes

The markers and symptoms of depression may be influenced and coloured by circumstances at the time. In this way a new episode of depression can arrive in disguise.

Lisa recalls:

When I was pregnant I felt great. Yes, I was tired and sore but I didn't feel any anxiety or concern about life with a new baby. I even recall mentioning to my GP that I was aware my history with depression would mean I was in a higher risk category for postnatal depression. But I had a plan and a supportive, loving family who knew the warning signs.

Looking back, it would seem I underestimated my depression and I forgot how clever I could be at masking the signs, even from myself. I think this is the surprising thing about depression. Inside you can be a mess and feel like the world is about to fall apart, but on the surface you're smiling, laughing and projecting the vision you so badly want to be the reality.

I suppose my first 'trigger' was that I didn't really get the three-day blues. At the time I thought it showed I was coping so well, I was going to skip the hormonal side of it all. Fantastic! But in reality it was a sign that I was already building walls around feelings that I thought weren't acceptable as a new parent. I hid it all away—even from myself.

Hilary describes panic attacks rather than a depressed mood as dominating after the birth of her third child:

My third encounter with postnatal depression was different from previous episodes. While the symptoms started at about the same time—ten days after giving birth—this time I was besieged by terrifying panic attacks. I would awaken during the night with my mind and body already engaged in a fully fledged attack. My heart would be racing, beating so hard and fast in my chest and in my ears that I thought I was surely having a heart attack.

Feeling down but calling it a difficult baby

Simone recounts her first inkling that her distress wasn't completely due to a fractious new baby. She titled her story 'Chicken and egg', noting that when she developed depression she was still a dreamy-eyed newlywed who never imagined the strain a baby would place on her and her marriage:

We have lovely photos of our life pre-baby, me doing my Bollywood best wrapped in a sari, gazing at my Indian prince. I had a genuine interest in my husband's culture—he had instilled it in me with stories of the village life which, as a new migrant, he was so homesick for. However, when it transpired that our baby was not a feed-and-sleep baby and when it further transpired that my husband would not be a hands-on father, all my enchantment disappeared. I just wanted someone to hold the baby so I could have a shower, someone to share my concern when our baby was diagnosed with silent reflux and failed to gain weight, someone to share the whole messy mess of it, good and bad. A night-shift worker, my husband would return home at 10 am, shower, sleep for a couple of hours, wake up and go to the gym or to visit friends. Anything, I guess, to escape the tearful twosome. Or rather, the tearful baby and the white-with-rage wife.

There is a photo, taken around Christmas 2006, when my son is about 6 weeks old—he is in the baby sling peering up at me and I am smiling wanly down at him. It looks like we are locked in a mother–child bonding moment, and we probably were, but if you look closer you can see that my eyes are red and puffy from crying, my hair scraped into a greasy, hasty ponytail, my skin a spotty mess. It could easily be a week since I'd last showered—he only slept in 20-minute snatches and I never seemed to get organised quickly enough. In fact, once he was finally asleep I would usually collapse into a chair, limp with bewilderment and exhaustion.

The first inkling I had that I may have had a problem occurred around this time. Once the baby had fed, and before he got tired and cranky, there was this lovely period of around half an hour where he would be a delightful, smiling, cooing little baby. The only problem was that during this happy 'awake' time, I would usually be crying. I would sit on the floor in front of him while he slouched casually in his bouncy-bub and I would sob and plead, beg him to be a better baby, to not cry so much, to sleep longer, to feed better, to not fuss at the breast and squirm away and scream, and please, please not cry so much. He would just keep gazing at me in that serene, curious way and one day I realised that, well, maybe the problem wasn't all him, maybe I was having some troubles of my own.

Of course, once I was diagnosed with postnatal depression (PND), things only got worse. For starters, my husband had never heard of it, insisted sniffily that no such thing existed in India, and as a result of my clumsy explanation of the condition, dismissed it as my 'hormone problem'. He was right about one thing, though: when I googled PND in India, all I got was an erroneous description of the baby blues that kick in for a few days after giving birth. Otherwise, there were references to research being undertaken on the subject, but nothing else.

When help is needed but the signals are missed

Naomi fooled herself and the midwives. She wrote that, from the first knowledge of her pregnancy, she started a 'grieving' process that lasted well into her son's first year. Her emotions ran amok. She'd cry for hours. Fears would grip her—of not being able to cope with daily mothering tasks and that she and her husband would be unable to support the baby:

I could feel acutely that a death and birth were taking place. The death of a free-spirited girl in her late 20s and the birth both of a mama and of a unique little person. I didn't know how to navigate the stormy seas of such change. I cursed myself for being overly sensitive

*about a natural transformation that was taking place. Why wasn't I
like the millions of mums that just 'got on with it' across the planet
and who were revelling in their pregnancy?*

*In hindsight my roller-coaster of emotions during pregnancy
should have triggered me to seek help before the birth but I was on a
quest to become the perfect mother. When midwives asked me how I
was feeling, I would shrug it off, 'Tired, a bit emotional, normal, you
know . . .'*

*Hark at this: sometimes it is all in the way a mother shrugs it off
that spells trouble.*

Sandra, in her essay titled 'Blue box' reflected on the possible tragic
consequences of her depression being missed. She judges that her
psychiatrist should have been contacted by the obstetric hospital
staff in the first week after her baby's birth. Sandra had had previous
psychiatric care and was, in a cursory way, under the care of a psychiatrist. But she observed:

*I don't think I was ever honest enough to tell anyone just how wrong
everything was becoming, because of my irrational fear that my baby
would be taken away. I think my husband and I both wanted to prove
that I was okay and that we could raise our baby like everyone else in
the world seemed to be able to do.*

*I have kept all the cards we were given when my son was born.
I still find them difficult to read, as I did back then. Packed away
in a small blue box, their joyful messages only serve to highlight the
absolute despair I felt after the birth of my baby. And, even now, a
twinge of shame still lingers.*

*Because of my history of depression, I kept watch over my moods
during my pregnancy. Yet I never felt any depression to report to the
prenatal psychiatrist during my two perfunctory appointments at
the hospital. The one thing I should have told her I did not, because
it terrified me so much that I denied to myself it had ever happened.
Once, when I was about six months pregnant and stopped at a red
light, I had the sudden urge to press my foot on the accelerator and
plough the car out into the passing traffic. It was a momentary thought*

that came from nowhere and left as soon as the lights changed. I drove on, shaking and disgusted at myself. I was protective of my bump. I loved my baby and my husband. That impulse at the traffic lights was that of a monster, wasn't it?

It was the first time I felt what would soon define my postnatal experience: shame and a deep fear that I was not normal. A fear that—despite the fact I was an articulate, functioning woman—if anyone knew just what I was feeling they would take my baby away. I would be like one of those women you read about in the newspaper.

After an induced and very long labour (he was 4.5 kilograms) I lay rigid in the hospital bed and began to lose my grip on reality, sliding into what felt like a parallel universe, observing my new self like a stranger and wondering where 'I' had gone. I watched in hazy detachment as my husband cared for the baby. I observed the midwife milk me like a dairy cow and feed the baby with a syringe, like those people you see on Animal Hospital *who rescue baby bats.*

On day 3 the psychiatrist came to see me briefly. She asked me if I felt depressed. I didn't feel detached from my baby, as I thought depressed mums did, so I said no. I did tell her I felt strange, like nothing was real and that I was very teary. She said I was right on schedule for the baby blues and it would probably pass. I was to start on antidepressants again, the dose I had been on before my pregnancy. The earliest follow-up psychiatric appointment that could be offered was five weeks away.

Privately, I started to wonder what the procedure was if a mother was too incompetent to look after her baby. I stopped being able to sleep and several times I broke down when a midwife casually asked me how I was going. They said it was good I had started medication. I was half-surprised when I was allowed to go home.

I know now that I was already succumbing to a postnatal mood disorder. However, my husband and I were on the lookout for 'depression'. I didn't feel depressed. I was, instead, in a constant state of high alert and borderline panic, barred from any sleep or rest by a mind that whirled nonstop with worries about feeding and sleeping times, child-safety hazards that wouldn't be relevant for months, schooling concerns that wouldn't be relevant for years.

Worst of all, every time I looked at my sleeping baby I saw myself placing my hand over his mouth. 'You're a monster,' I said to myself. Again I told no one. I thought if anyone knew what was in my head they would take my baby away. Even now I want to make it clear I didn't want to hurt my baby.

I refused to get someone to come and help me during the day, because that just wasn't what people did. I could only sleep for 45 minutes at most, even when the baby was asleep. If someone visited I would have to dress and brush my teeth. I would have to make tea and wash up the mugs after they left. I would have to smile and laugh like new mothers who are in love with their babies do.

My husband was wonderfully patient and supportive of me, but we both felt there was nothing that could be done. (We now also recognise that he had slid into depression himself; the pressure of working a 50-hour week and holding everything together at home had become overwhelming.) I was already on medication. I had told my GP at the check-up that I didn't want to go home. She responded that I needed to relax. She assumed the hospital psychiatrist had it under control. She told me I couldn't take sleep medication because I was breastfeeding. She told me to have a drink of warm milk before bed.

Well, we didn't make it to the five-week psychiatric follow-up. The sense that there was nothing more that could be done for me drove me very close to suicide one morning not long after my husband had returned to work. Again without any sleep, I felt utterly overwhelmed by the day ahead and was prepared to do anything to stop the endless obsessive cycle in my head. I stood staring at the knife block and I still thank God every day that it was the phone I picked up that morning and not a knife. I rang my mother and told her I needed help. I was too ashamed to ring my husband. I didn't want to let him down.

The local adult mental health crisis team intervened. The social worker asked me if I had ever thought of harming myself or my baby. It is impossible to own up to something so shameful when your partner is sitting right next to you. But when I saw another psychiatrist a week later it was the first time I felt safe enough to admit just how bad things were in my head.

Without private health insurance, the fees at the private hospital mother-and-baby unit were well out of our reach. Tresillian was booked out. The hospital had no beds for a mother and baby. My husband took time off work, and the baby bonus and friends helped us pay the rent. I began months of sedation and medication switches as my psychiatrist searched for a solution to my anxiety.

Looking back . . . what would have helped:
- *I believe it is vital that new mothers be assured that every effort will be made to keep them with their baby—no matter what. I was desperately afraid of what would happen if I told someone how I truly felt.*
- *The term 'postnatal depression' was also misleading to me. What I experienced was unlike any depression I had ever endured before, only enforcing the idea that there was something fundamentally wrong with me.*
- *It is also imperative to remove any fears women may have about relying on medication. Antidepressants didn't bother me, it was sedatives and antipsychotics and tranquillisers that convinced me I would surely become an addict and made me feel I had a deadline I must recover by. This wasn't helped by one counsellor who told me she didn't believe in medication and that it was probably making me suicidal.*
- *I was terrified I would never be myself again—never get my mind back. That was how sick I had become. I asked my psychiatrist over and over if I would ever get better. I would have benefited from access to stories of survival and recovery: the DVDs I was shown all focused on understanding the signs of postnatal depression—testimonies of experience, but not recovery.*

Now, nearly three years later . . .
Now my son is the greatest joy I have ever known and I thoroughly enjoy motherhood. Most of the medication has been replaced by regular exercise—my three swimming sessions a week are non-negotiable in our household.

My husband and I want more children, but I am still shaken after my experience. In the meantime I am learning to forgive myself, and learning to read those cards and not feel shame.

No recognition of what the problem might be

I know the signs and symptoms of depression. I am a midwife, so this is part of my training. And I have suffered from depression before. So I have experienced depression from both sides of the black shadow. As a midwife I know the importance of answering the postnatal depression questionnaire honestly. Well, I ticked all the boxes and scored as healthy. Now I know I was not honest; not on purpose, just unknowingly. I wanted to enjoy that special pregnancy bubble that so many people talk about. Well, depression came out of nowhere and blew me and my family away for four long years.

Jane

Marcie described how she was able to disguise her numbness and lack of feelings, until disabling anxiety made it impossible to feign 'normal' reactions any longer. She observed how endless darkness followed her around, coming in waves. She had lost herself and her once-optimistic rose-coloured glasses; she couldn't even find the energy to look for them. She had no notion that she was experiencing PND until faced with the disabling anxiety that began to accompany her depression.

I watched my husband feed my little baby girl and knew that they shared the bond that was supposed to be mine. I felt no maternal instincts, no yearnings and no special connection. Could I buy a bottle of that from the chemist perhaps? But I couldn't ask over the counter because what sort of person am I not to have motherly feelings towards my baby? I think I was ashamed and very disappointed in myself. I felt I had got myself into something that was completely beyond me and I was failing miserably.

Solution. In public, be perfect, well adjusted. Smile when required, ooh and ahh when appropriate, carry a camera and don't leave the baby in the car park at the supermarket. At home, break down uncontrollably, wish your life was back to how it was 12 months ago, abuse husband and watch loads of television. And this worked, for a little while at least.

Until the anxiety set in.

Since when was going for a walk an issue? Why couldn't I go on a train without passing out? Why couldn't I travel a kilometre from home without my stomach knotting? And the phone, surely we could disconnect it so I didn't have to talk to anybody? When did the daily trip to the letterbox become my only outing? And the panic attacks!

Thus began regular trips to the local GP. Then the pills, my 'happy pills'. Then the visits to the shrink. Now, that was an issue. Firstly I had to drive 60 kilometres. And see a shrink? What the . . .? How embarrassing. I'm not a nut job. What if this gets out? Will I lose my job? Will people look at me funny when I walk down the street? Do I have to wear a bracelet?

What it actually meant was self-examination, awareness, acknowledgment, hope. A change of pills. Finally, stuff started making sense. My life was regaining focus. That massive big black hole that was my world now had a door. The door was locked, mind you, and distant, but it was there. And that mattered. I could work towards something without dread and suffocating hopelessness.

It's been an arduous journey and there are days when I slip. But there are days now when life is so sweet I get a toothache. I know that I will have to remain vigilant—that is my lot. But now I know how to do it. And I am damn proud to say that now I have three beautiful girls; all priceless gifts that I would commit to again—without hesitation. The bond I share with each one is my own personal cure for my not-so-great days.

Jodie described her mood disorder as more of a 'numb state'. For her, public spaces and socialising, which depressed people often avoid because they find them stressful, provided a partially helpful coping strategy:

When my husband was at work, I was alone. Alone with the children. I reverted to a numb, zombie state. I could hardly respond to them and when I did it seemed to be in slow motion. I couldn't smile. I couldn't laugh with my beautiful little boy as he was giggling away and dancing with the Wiggles on the video. I was fearful of my inability to fully respond and care for them. And I feared anyone finding out.

I read that many women experiencing postnatal depression have difficulty leaving the house. Well I had difficulty staying home. I didn't know what was wrong with me but I did know that the only way I could force myself to care for my children was to be in public. In public I was motivated by fear of failure and judgement. In public I cared for my children. So I wandered shopping centres and parks for hours. I visited neighbours and fellow mothers from mothers' group—anything to force myself to care for the little ones.

One day I found myself in mothers' group, surrounded by people talking and laughing and then the sounds became blurry. I could only stare: time seemed to slow down, everything was in slow motion, I felt frozen, I couldn't move, I couldn't respond, I felt empty. I felt alone, so very alone and lonely, in a room full of people. It terrified me. This depressive state had now found me in public.

No one ever spoke of postnatal depression. It seemed to be a no-go zone, a taboo. They all kept their happy masks on, saying they loved parenting and healthy routines and habits. The focus of conversation always went towards children and babies, never ourselves.

SEEKING HELP AND REAPING THE BENEFITS

A disabling low mood in a pregnant woman or a new (or not-so-new) mother can be missed because it can be easy to disguise distress, even from yourself, in the limited time of a visit to the GP, the antenatal check-up or while the baby is being weighed.

Helen put on a brave face, too. She didn't seek treatment when she was diagnosed with PND . . . at first. Besides, she didn't believe the diagnosis related to her. Sometimes she was fine. She didn't think anyone could help her anyway. She didn't need more pressure and lists of things she should do—she lacked the time. So she pushed on until her breaking point and then recognised the consequences of her untreated mood disorder.

She observes:

I came home from the doctor and said to my husband, 'Postnatal depression?' and he didn't believe it. He hadn't seen it. I was all right when he was around. It was when I was alone, when no one was watching, that I broke down. I was unsure of the diagnosis myself. I thought being depressed meant you always walked around crying. Sometimes I was fine. When I got out of the house and managed to escape I felt calm and peaceful. Although now diagnosed with depression, I felt like a fake, like a fraud, as though I wasn't entitled to being unwell and asking for help.

I didn't think anyone could really help me anyway. Doctor visits meant long hours in crowded waiting rooms with hungry, tantrum-throwing kids who needed to use the toilet and fought over the one sticky toy by the magazines. It was hard enough without seeking punishment like that. And therapy? I'd never been to therapy. What could they tell me that I didn't already know? That I wasn't already trying to do? I didn't need more pressure. I didn't need more lists of things I should do for which I didn't have the energy.

One day I snapped. We were late going somewhere, probably to the doctor, and my son wouldn't put on his shoes. I still had the baby to feed, hats to find and nappies to check. I'd asked him a dozen times. So I screamed at him. Crazy, psycho-lady scream. 'GET YOUR SHOES ON NOW!' I was rough with him as I pulled his leg up and thrust his sandal on. I continued shouting . . . Then I looked up and by chance my eyes met his.

How to describe what I saw in that moment? I saw my baby boy, now a big boy. I saw his beautiful brown eyes, pained and hurt. I saw how he wouldn't look at me, but stared out the window. I saw the stubborn set to his jaw and sensed the strength of his little soul, that even when shouted at by a lunatic, he knew who he was and that he was of worth. And I asked myself, 'What am I doing?' I am this wonderful little boy's mother. Mine is the name he calls when sick or afraid. Mine are the arms he wants to hold him, to reassure him that he is loved. I am the tickler, the giggler, the one who can build the tallest tower out of Duplo. I am his mother. I'm supposed to be his champion, his hero, the one who believes in him and helps him face the outside world. What am I doing, shrieking at him, screaming at him, out of control? What must he be thinking? How must he be feeling when so abused by the mother he loves?

I felt a sob rise through me as I put my arms around his little body, pulling him to my chest. 'I'm sorry, so sorry. You don't deserve to be shouted at. Mummy shouldn't shout at you. You're a good boy. I love you, I love you.' And that's when I knew I needed help.

I called my doctor and found a babysitter for the appointment. I didn't feel guilty. I would sail the world and climb the highest mountain if my son needed me. And my son needed me to go to my doctor. So I went. I pushed my fears of medication aside. I'd tried to do this on my own for so long, now it was time to trust someone else. It was time to ask for help. So I accepted the medication.

I saw an advert for a group therapy session and I scribbled the details on the back of a dry cleaner's receipt. I called that afternoon. I attended every single session, never missing one. I even went on bad days, when my hair was a mess and I was running late and shouting at my kids, because my children needed me to go on those days most of all. And for them, I would do anything, even go to therapy in disarray.

The medication helped. The load lightened. I took my kids for a walk one day by choice and I enjoyed it. I watched them laugh and run and play and I took pleasure in it all. I noticed that the sun was shining. Sometimes I felt down again. Sometimes I got too busy and tried to do too much and then a dark shadow fell over me, even with the medication. With therapy, I was able to think about that, to discuss it and seek answers about the why. And then anticipate or strive to minimise it.

I still see a counsellor and I'm still on medication, but I've learned so much to help me on my way. I have come to understand myself, how my body works and how my thoughts run, in an astonishingly intimate and unique way. And I realise that having postnatal depression isn't a weakness, but an opportunity to gain strength. It's not something I am ashamed of. Instead, I feel I deserve an award, a badge pinned to my chest stating to everyone where I have been and how far I have come.

I am not weak because I have postnatal depression. I am a champion because I got help.

Recognising an illness and being prepared

Sometimes the speed of events overtakes us before we're prepared. There seems to be no time to adapt to too many changes at once. As Darcy says in her story, titled 'Road to recovery', 'Wow. That was fast.' Everything was going according to plan, except it all felt wrong.

Darcy developed a very severe depressive illness. She isolated herself and, though desperately lonely, avoided almost all social contact, feeling that she couldn't be 'normal' and that any sort of conversation would give her away. By this time, she says, 'I was living in a strange, muffled, black-and-white world, peopled by myself, my son and my mind.' She became panicky, obsessive and suicidal.

But during her next pregnancy she was prepared. She was fortunate to find a counsellor who diagnosed her severe mood swings as part of a bipolar II disorder (see Chapter 1). There is a vital message in Darcy's account. Sometimes a mood disorder is precipitated or unveiled by the changes, including hormonal fluctuations, occurring during pregnancy, childbirth and the demands of the early months of motherhood, particularly sleeplessness. The symptoms and signs of bipolar disorder are listed in Chapter 1, and an anonymous self-test is available on the Black Dog Institute website.[2]

Darcy recounts the speed of events and their consequences:

'Congratulations, you got the job!'

I gave the thumbs up signal to my husband.

'When can you start?'

'I'm actually in the car driving to Wagga now,' I laughed. 'So, any time!'

Our tree change was off to a good start. We were leaving our much loved but expensive suburb of Sydney for a large country town. I'd spent my childhood in a small town nearby, and was hoping to recapture the happiness I'd felt amidst the rolling hills. Our plan was to get jobs, buy a house, start a family, and live happily ever after. So far so good. If I'd had any idea of what we were actually heading into, I would have screamed for my husband to turn the car around. But instead we kept driving, oblivious to the yawning black hole ahead.

'Congratulations! You're pregnant!'
Wow. That was fast. One month into my new job and I'm trying to hide the nausea. Still, you can't order a baby and we had friends who had been trying to conceive for years, so we knew we were incredibly lucky.

'Sold!'
Two months later, we were in our new house. Everything was going to plan. Except it all felt wrong. This region was supposed to be my home, but I felt like a stranger. Had we made a wrong turn? I could feel my dream sliding away. I was due to go on maternity leave soon and I had made no real friends. A sense of foreboding settled upon me.

'It's a boy!'
I loved my son instantly. But with that love came something else completely unexpected. Fear. I held my tiny son and was engulfed by fear.

Our son!
He was beautiful, but he cried. I walked around the house for hours, trying to rock him to sleep. I took the night shift alone because we were worried that my husband, a builder, would injure himself at work if he was too tired. Plus I could sleep during the day when the baby did. Except my son rarely slept in his bed, preferring to sleep in my arms as I walked. In addition to extreme fatigue, I was beginning to feel incredibly lonely. I began to dread the night shift and would feel anxious and afraid by 3 pm. But I was too ashamed to tell anyone how I was feeling. I was a mother! Motherhood is the most wonderful experience of a woman's life, right?

The days and nights blurred together. I lived in my pyjamas. I went to bed in a stupor, only to wake an hour later. I played little games,

*collecting times of interest on the digital clock beside the bed: 1.11 am,
2.22 am, 3.33 am.*

*One night, I was passing through the kitchen on my well-worn
circuit, crying son in my arms, when a sudden rage engulfed me. I felt
an urge to swing him through the air and smash him into the bench
to stop the noise. 'I just need you to SHUT. UP.' Then there would be
silence. Then I could sleep. Then this nightmare would be over.*

*The fury dissipated, leaving me beyond horrified. Crying, I hugged
his little body and fled from the room. I continued my circuit at a
rapid rate, trying to calm myself. Each time I passed through the
kitchen, I could see the bench in my peripheral vision. Was I going to
do it this time? Or this time? Eventually I avoided the kitchen, pacing
through the living room, on the verge of waking my husband. But
what would I tell him? Fear and panic set in. That I wanted to murder
my child? But I loved him! What was happening to me?*

*The next evening, I told my husband. I could barely meet his gaze.
He looked at me as if seeing a stranger, and after a long silence said,
'If you ever hurt him . . .'*

*'I know,' I said. 'I would never hurt him. I know that.' But I had
lost my self-trust. I had no idea who I was anymore.*

*Out of desperation, I joined a mothers' group. I would sit and chat,
surreptitiously studying the other women for signs of distress. One girl
was obviously suffering, her tear-stained face drawing sympathy from
the group. I avoided her. I was used to being a success and wanted pity
from no one. So I did my utmost to act 'normal'. It was exhausting.*

*At home, things were going downhill. I cried every day. I had panic
attacks about my son's safety, fearing he would be kidnapped. I gave
myself pep talks to make it to the clothes line and back while he slept
inside. The baby monitor was useless because I feared someone could
jump the fence, sneak inside silently, spirit him away.*

*I became fixated on his temperature and got out of bed constantly
to add or remove blankets. I checked the locks obsessively: 'Did I
lock the laundry door? I can't remember, I'd better go check. Ah
yes, it's locked.' Twenty minutes later: 'Did I lock the laundry door?
I think so, but maybe I'm remembering locking it last night. Better
go check . . .'*

My tolerance for his crying diminished to almost nothing and I would quickly become enraged. Many times I had to put him down somewhere safe and walk away to calm myself. I never, ever, hurt him, but the fear that I would was constant. It gradually dawned on me that the biggest threat to my beloved son's safety wasn't the kidnappers over the back fence. It was me. His mother. The day I realised that was perhaps the saddest day of my life.

I fantasised about suicide. My son would be better off without me and my husband could marry a happy woman. But I couldn't deny that my breastmilk was doing him good. Often it was the only positive thing I could think of that I could provide for him. Okay, I'd finish breastfeeding him and then I'd kill myself. As traumatic as the thought was, I needed to know I had a way out.

Once suicide became an almost daily thought I finally knew I needed help. I had three visits to two different psychologists, to no avail. I hadn't found the right person. But I knew I had to act. I began to open up to my husband and my mother. We taught our son to settle himself and I began exercising and repeating endless positive affirmations. I whispered a promise in my son's little ear that I would do whatever it took to get better.

When my son was 6 months old, I went back to work, my husband taking on the role of full-time carer. I continued breastfeeding. Rejoining the workforce was my salvation. I was part of the community again. I gradually became a version of my former self, albeit shell-shocked.

'Congratulations, you're pregnant!'

When our son was 15 months old we tried for another baby. One month later I was pregnant. I was happy, but anxious. So this time we asked for help. I swallowed my pride and told my parents, my obstetrician and close friends that I'd suffered from postnatal depression. I became increasingly anxious and depressed as the due date loomed over the horizon like a dark cloud, ready to engulf me again. I arranged to see yet another psychologist, and thankfully we clicked. The difference was immense. I felt like a boxer exhausted from a long, lonely fight whose coach had finally appeared.

'It's a girl!'
This time things were different. My husband and family rallied. I had my 'coach' and, in a poignant turn, my son kept me company. My husband helped me at night, and we taught our daughter to self-settle almost immediately. Now my daughter is 4 months old and we're doing well. I still battle with mood swings and the same obsessive behaviours but I don't feel alone anymore.

'I think there's a possibility you have a bipolar II disorder.'
After the initial shock of a psychiatrist's diagnosis, I'm beginning to feel a sense of relief. Finally, I might get some answers about why I am the way I am and learn to live a happier life.

The road we drove down took some unexpected turns, but I now have two beautiful children, my husband and I are closer than ever, and together we'll keep travelling to recovery.

Perhaps I wouldn't turn the car around after all.

Accepting permission to drop the mask

Lisa adopted an 'everything's under control' mask: if her home was clean and tidy and dinner organised by 5.30 pm it showed the world that there was nothing wrong, she was coping, and she was a competent wife and mother. But she felt, deep down, that nothing she did was enough, especially when it came to their baby. She covered up her profound belief that she was a failure as a mother, that everything she did was wrong, and that it was only a matter of time before her husband and family discovered what a 'hopeless fraud' she was.

In a contrasting scenario, Hilary describes the immense relief she experienced when the social worker she met gave her the time and approval to drop her mask. In such an accepting environment she felt safe and could abandon the exhausting charade of imitating how a 'good mother' would look after her baby:

From my first meeting with the social worker I was convinced this woman was my saving angel. She sat me down and let me cry quietly, totally unperturbed by my tears. This woman educated me about postnatal depression—an illness I had now been diagnosed with but knew nothing about in terms of treatment and prognosis. I still cannot find words to describe the sense and depth of relief I felt upon meeting her.

What followed was a year of weekly visits where I could gradually start to speak of my feelings, my despair and my pain. There was no judgement. There was no telling me to 'pull your socks up and just get on with it'. No talk about the 'right way' to do everything. From this woman came acceptance and a reassuring confidence that I would eventually recover—and that how I was managing meanwhile was better than I could perceive.

Shamilla credited 'the keen eye and astute mind' of her maternal health centre sister with the recognition that something was wrong. About five weeks after the birth she picked up the signs. She suggested that Shamilla attend a group where women having difficulties were offered a supportive environment. Shamilla was apprehensive, as she was rather shy and the thought of sitting among a group of women who she was sure had more confidence than she did was intimidating:

Despite this, something in the back of my mind said, 'DO IT!' I would later come to realise that instinct is often silenced by the chattering voice of negativity.

I recall, when attending my first group meeting, feeling normal for the first time since the birth. I was 'normal' amongst these amazing women, as long as I was with them. When I'd step back into the outside world it was then that I felt dysfunctional. I couldn't wait to reunite with them the following week.

It was within this group that I had my epiphany, the one that changed my life forever. As the facilitator asked us for the typical traits of our depression, I came to study the whiteboard she wrote upon: anger, sadness, lethargy, resentment, obsessive control (the oppressor), hopelessness . . . Instead of beating ourselves up over these things we found we were laughing about how much we had in common, telling stories regarding our long-suffering partners.

As the list went on so did a switch in my mind. I was suddenly given the opportunity to see who I was not. All these traits did not belong to me; they belonged to the depression itself or what I like to refer to as 'the demon and its cape'. Naked (so to speak), I was me, the real me. As soon as I could see the illness through my new eyes I envisaged this hideous beast holding onto a heavy black cape with words like 'loser', 'useless', 'burden', 'hopeless', 'failure', pinned to it. It had enveloped me and this was the persona I saw every time I looked at myself—questioning my purpose for being here ('Such a waste of space,' I'd thought).

Finally the cape had been removed, my demon was gone, no longer whispering lies into my ear, and I felt light. Underneath I was not the person who belonged to the horrible labels. I was me, the wide-eyed child with a passion for life and a view of a beautiful world, re-energised and starting out afresh.

The roadblocks to seeking care

Our writers have related poignant and harrowing stories of their experiences with PND, as well as factors that prevented or delayed their awareness of the condition or prevented them from feeling comfortable about seeking help. It is clear from such accounts (admittedly weighted to those with the most severe conditions) that there are many roadblocks to awareness and seeking help for a post-natal mood disorder.

So many women viewed their distress as a failure rather than an illness. Additionally, depression 'talks'. One mother said, 'When you're down you just can't see any options, but the minute your mood lifts you can see that there are choices and that you can take action.' Many women were also unable to understand whether their distress was part of adjustment to motherhood or whether it was depression or an anxiety disorder. Many denied their distress (even to themselves) because of worry about where a diagnosis might lead and its consequences. And most were unsure at which point they should seek help.

BARRIERS TO SEEKING HELP

beyondblue, the Australian national depression initiative, has issued guidelines relating to depression in the perinatal period. They summarise the main reasons why mothers don't seek help, even when they've run out of reserves and feel dangerously near the edge.

Barriers that prevent or inhibit women from seeking help include:[3]

- *Knowledge barriers*—women believe their symptoms of distress are a normal part of motherhood. They are unable to distinguish between normal levels of distress and distress that warrants help, or they don't know where to seek help.
- *Attitude barriers*—including reluctance to disclose emotional problems to health professionals (women feel they should be able to cope on their own and/or do not want to be a burden), lack of motivation to seek treatment, fear of stigma and fear of losing the baby and/or other children if diagnosed with a mental health disorder. Women may also minimise or hide symptoms to preserve an image of themselves as competent mothers.
- *Service barriers*—including women's concerns about unhelpful responses from health providers (such as their feelings being dismissed or trivialised), negative prior experiences with or lack of trust in care providers, concerns about privacy and confidentiality, and unwillingness to take antidepressant medication.
- *Logistical barriers*—including lack of time, problems finding child care, cost of treatment, transport problems and long waiting times for appointments.

Pride is another huge barrier: many women feel a loss of face if they admit to suffering from depression. They consider it a weakness, not a treatable problem.

eight

Where to get help

Life is like a journey across the country. Sometimes your car breaks down and you need help. Likewise, the therapist needs to find where you are and help you from there. They may be able to take you a short distance or a long distance, but starting to move is the main thing, along with accepting when you are all right on your own again.

Samira

SUPPORT IS ESSENTIAL—AND SUCH A RELIEF

Support is critically important. Before we look at the assistance that can be provided by health professionals for a new family, it's worth mentioning what's available closer to home. Family and friends can and want to provide help.

There are different types of support:
- *Practical support* could be baby-related (bathing or feeding the baby) or non-baby-related (washing up, shopping or providing a meal).
- *Social support* includes the gift of companionship of the type and at the time wanted by the new family.
- *Emotional support*, so essential for new mothers, revolves around sharing positive events (baby has just smiled) as well as negative ones (baby has enduring tummy problems).

Perhaps the most important source of this support is your partner—particularly given that research shows an unsupportive partner is the strongest risk factor for PND.[1] Your own mother and her partner's mother can be key sources of support. One caveat ... groundwork may be necessary: mothers and mothers-in-law can be critical or perceived to be judgemental. This can be a trigger for PND, or perpetuate it.

Good help can be hard to find

Help is not always readily available, let alone affordable or suitable. Our essayists were more likely to describe difficulties rather than a smooth track to assistance. We provide examples of some contrasting pathways and outcomes.

Judy describes an unfortunately all-too-common situation as she recounts her first antenatal visit. It's an outback doctor's surgery and she is a new mother, her baby only 6 weeks old. Her husband, having driven her and the baby 150 kilometres to see the doctor, cradles the little girl, their first child.

She titled her experience, 'A first-time mother: the rural perspective'. The doctor asks why they are there:

'I was told to see my doctor for a check-up after six weeks.'

'Ohh?' (A casual reply.) 'Uh, well, how are you?'

'Still in a lot of pain. The caesarean scar doesn't seem to be healing properly.'

'Well, it's a bit early to worry. Everything else okay?'

(Her records on his computer should remind him that she has suffered from depression in the past.)

'Hmm, I'm actually not too good in my head.'

'Well yes!' (Uncomfortable laugh.) 'No one is, with a new baby!'

'But I keep reliving the birth, and I cry all the time. We've talked quite often with the breastfeeding helpline and I think we finally know how to feed her, but I keep wanting not to be here, and sometimes to throw her out the window too.'

'Well, that's pretty much how every new mum feels. Try to get some sleep when she does.'

'But she only sleeps for 20 minutes or so at a time—surely that's not right for a tiny baby?'

(Uncomfortable laugh.) 'Mmmm, some kids just don't sleep much! Now, we'll see you in two weeks to look her over and give her the first lot of needles.'

'Aren't you going to check my scar?'

'It's probably fine. Come back if it still hurts.'

Dismissed, the young couple head home feeling more lost and alone. In the long months that follow, it was only their desperate desire to be parents and an attitude of 'us against the world' that got them through. Having been through a miscarriage already, they knew heartbreak and grief and they had survived by clinging to each other, and they instinctively did that again.

Being on an isolated property, with few visitors and even fewer chances to socialise, they found help online, from the Australian Breast-feeding Association and other websites. They fought and they argued, but kept to their vow to always talk to each other. The husband would turn up at home early just to check on his 'two girls', and he learned to put up with mood swings, or to hold a screaming baby while his wife sought a short refuge outdoors. He was a man who would do anything for his wife and he was a dad who would do anything for his daughter.

And, as she got more sleep and baby responded more she felt a bit better. As time went by and they learned how to be parents it brought fulfilment that overrode the sacrifices. And gradually she could take pleasure in the little things, a tiny hand curled against her neck . . .

And so the young couple decided to have a second baby. After a further two miscarriages, he arrived alive and healthy, and the over-joyed mother was on a natural high for weeks. The quick recovery from a natural delivery, and the empowerment from this birth (the midwife for the first baby had been so discouraging and worse than unhelpful) delighted both parents. Even sex was again joyful instead of fraught with pain and fearful memories. The mother's moods were more stable and she was calmer. But eventually the euphoria lapsed. She rang Lifeline and got a counsellor who was fabulous and who would ring her so that she didn't have to drag two little ones into town every few weeks.

Now the (not-so-young-anymore) couple have their third baby. Circumstances had changed pretty dramatically. My husband had returned to his previous job to supplement the family's income as the drought had been ongoing for many years. After the excellent counsellor left the district, the new one was not so good a match. But we knew that I needed one to keep me going and after a few months I found one who matches me fabulously. She describes my workload as 'humanly impossible'—I run the property on my own while my husband works away, and I started teaching one child last year—yet I'm still alive. (Ridiculously, I am now afraid of dying—after sometimes fantasising that suicide would be the best answer, now that seems ironic!)

These days I am mindful of giving myself some 'me' time and some 'husband and me' time—even though it can be so hard when you are a long way from babysitters or day care. But most of all (and hardest) is to accept that there is a physical reason for me not being 'normal'. I still fall into the trap of thinking it's my own personality or my own fault that my head lets me down. I still struggle to accept that there is nothing wrong with me as a person, that it is a disorder of my brain chemistry.

And we hope that somehow there's a way our struggle can be of benefit to others. I also hope I can help my children learn that mental illness doesn't have to ruin your life, even though it will rule the way you live.

The relief of confiding in someone who cares

Nadia felt that she had brought mental torture on herself by daring to have a baby; she deserved it. 'This was my punishment—a life sentence, motherhood—just for being me.' One day, about four months after giving birth, she found herself sitting on the cold bathroom tiles holding a razor in her hand that she had absolutely no idea what she was going to do with . . . The shock of this gave her perspective on how far she had slipped:

Who had I become? And why? I did not want to die—but I just did not want to exist anymore. There was no way out. What was the reward for all this? Suddenly it was all too hard. I was exhausted.

My husband encouraged me to see my GP and implored me to be honest. In tears, I told my doctor that I just couldn't see the light at the end of the tunnel, that I wanted the ground to open up and swallow me.

Gently and compassionately, he explained that it was not my fault, that I was doing nothing wrong. What a relief! Right there and then, I felt the weight sliding from my shoulders.

After questioning me about my support networks and devising a mental health plan, he recommended some ongoing counselling, urging me to reach out for support and to stop hiding how I felt. He also prescribed a low-dosage antidepressant—something not contraindicated with breastfeeding—and supported me in my decision that weaning was just not an option I would consider.

After about two weeks of taking the medication I started to notice a difference. Glimmers of light were appearing at the edges of my thoughts—I just had to try. The counsellor gave me perspective, too. There now seemed time for me to shower each day, to brush my teeth and do my hair. It was okay to smile and laugh because sometimes, things were worth smiling about.

And I recovered fully and now pass on this salutary tale to you.

WHO CAN HELP?

Here is a list of some sources of help suggested by women with a perinatal mood disorder. Health professionals of the same discipline may have very different treatment styles. If you find you're not compatible with a particular person or they make you feel judged or uncomfortable, it's perfectly all right to seek out another.

- A *childcare nurse* or *mothercraft nurse* from the baby health clinic. Mothercraft nurses are specially trained in all aspects of labour, newborns and child care. They can be particularly helpful for primary stresses such as difficulty in feeding or settling the baby, or worries about what is or isn't normal for a newborn.
- *Social workers* can be helpful in linking families and mothers to appropriate services and resources. As well as knowing about regional community and assistance groups, they can provide

information and support for the growing family and counselling or even parenting skills training.

- A wise family *GP* is a great place to start. Many are comfortable managing a woman with a perinatal disorder (including prescribing medication, providing advice on managing the new baby and alleviating anxieties about the physical health of both), and they can also provide referrals to other health professionals such as psychiatrists and psychologists.

- *Psychologists* and *clinical psychologists* both provide psychotherapy, the difference being that clinical psychologists will have completed an additional postgraduate course at university. The most common form of therapy currently practised by psychologists is cognitive behavioural therapy (CBT), which identifies and addresses thoughts and behaviours that trigger or prolong low moods. A competent psychologist can tailor therapy to your needs and experiences.

- *Psychiatrists* have undergone extensive medical training and specialised in mental health. A psychiatrist should be able to determine what treatment approach is optimal and, if medication is necessary, to prescribe and monitor treatment. A subset of *perinatal psychiatrists* specialise in treating mental health issues during or following pregnancy and can provide the best information about medications during pregnancy and breast-feeding if these are needed.

- *Counsellors* can be useful to help you understand problems and come up with effective solutions. They may also help with difficulties you or your partner may have in adjusting to your new roles. 'Counsellor' is a generic term adopted by a variety of people who offer assistance. Ensure that your chosen counsellor has professional qualifications and skills you feel confident with.

- *Private hospitals* and *private psychiatric clinics* have a range of professionals available for consultation. Many also offer specialised education programs and support groups.

- Your *local hospital* or *area mental health service* will have an outpatient facility with variable capacity for assessing and assisting women with a perinatal condition.

- Your local hospital's *emergency department* can provide assessment in a crisis. There are also *emergency telephone counselling services*, such as Lifeline (13 11 14).
- In most large cities *multicultural services* can provide counsellors to assist women who are not English speakers and have an understanding of cultural and background nuances. Such staff can also act as interpreters, and they provide services to all major hospitals. Start your search with Multicultural Mental Health Australia (website listed below).
- A number of organisations—such as *Tresillian* and *Karitane*—provide parenting advice to mothers and families and also have residential facilities. Such facilities, because they are not a mental health service, can provide a less confronting experience and allay concerns about being seen to have a mental illness.
- There are many helpful *websites*, including (listed alphabetically):

Australian Breastfeeding Association: www.breastfeeding.asn.au
beyondblue: www.beyondblue.org.au/resources/for-me/
    pregnancy-and-early-parenthood
Black Dog Institute: www.blackdoginstitute.org.au/public/
    depression/inpregnancypostnatal/babyblues.cfm
Gidget Foundation: www.gidgetfoundation.com.au
Good Beginnings: www.goodbeginnings.org.au
Karitane: www.karitane.com.au/index.php
Lifeline: www.lifeline.org.au
Men's Line Australia: www.mensline.org.au
Mental Health in Multicultural Australia: www.mhima.org.au
Parent–Infant Research Institute: www.piri.org.au/index.php
Parent Link: www.parentlink.act.gov.au
Post and Antenatal Depression Association: www.panda.org.au
Pregnancy, Birth and Baby Helpline, 1800 882 436: www.
    pregnancybirthbaby.org.au
Tresillian: www.tresillian.net
What Were We Thinking!: www.whatwerewethinking.org.au/
    index.php

THE INGREDIENTS OF AN IDEAL ASSESSMENT

Background information

Before or following initial assessment, the health professional should be prepared to receive information if contacted by a worried relative but not to transmit any personal information or clinical assessment details to that person without your specific permission.

Content

In an ideal assessment, the health professional determines whether depression is your main disorder or a consequence of another primary condition (such as anxiety or physical problems). If your depression is significant, the professional should determine its key features in order to determine the subtype, upon which treatment and management approaches will depend, and work out to what degree the illness is impairing your ability to function. They should enquire about your coping skills, risk factors and recent history.

Risk assessment

This should cover your possible thoughts of self-harm and/or thoughts of harming the baby or yourself. As well, the assessment should cover your genetic risk (whether you have a family history of mood problems), triggers to the episode (such as a difficult birth, a hard-to-settle baby, isolation), predisposing factors (such as anxiety, perfectionism) and perpetuating factors (such as financial difficulties, problems with your partner). Your life history of depressive episodes and mood swings, and previous treatments and their effectiveness (or ineffectiveness), will not only provide important information but also help narrow treatment options. Any medical or surgical problems should be noted, as well as allergies—especially to medications—and any history of drug and alcohol use.

Family and background

The health professional should seek to learn more about your life: your family background; how you were parented; whether you experienced stressors such as bullying or abuse during your earlier years; your career; the quality of your current intimate, family and peer relationships; and, in particular, your views about being a mother and about your baby.

What to expect

At assessment you should expect confidentiality, empathy, under-standing and enough time to express your thoughts and feelings. While it can often help the health practitioner to obtain further information from a relative, you should feel free to ask the practitioner to respect your confidentiality. The assessment should lead to a provisional diagnosis, postulates about causes and a management plan. It is often helpful to allow a key family member to join the discussion about management plan details—especially who is to be responsible for what.

HARM, SELF-HARM AND INTRUSIVE THOUGHTS ASSOCIATED WITH PND

Any woman with a perinatal mood disorder should expect a risk assessment. Although discomfiting for everyone, it is a responsibility placed on a health professional. The assessment of PND considers the level of support and security needed by the mother and baby (which doctors call the dyad) if and while the mother's judgement is impaired.

A significant percentage of mothers experiencing PND have intrusive thoughts of harming their baby or that the baby will come to harm. Having read the accounts in this book, you may have been surprised how prevalent thoughts like these are. In reality, such obsessional thoughts are rarely acted upon. Many mothers get frustrated or resentful of their baby at times and may have angry thoughts towards it (especially when the infant 'refuses' to go to sleep). The words of the timeless nursery rhyme 'Rock-a-bye baby' hint at this ambivalence.

Obsessive thoughts can also be a symptom of obsessive-compulsive disorder (OCD), an anxiety disorder noted in Chapter 1. Obsessions in OCD are completely out of character with the sufferer's personality (professionals call this 'ego alien'). A clinical assessment will pursue whether you have such thoughts and, if so, whether they're part of OCD or a symptom of your depressive state. The good news is that there are techniques to control such thoughts. On occasion, especially if you are experiencing puerperal psychosis (see Chapter 1), such ruminations can indicate heightened risk that calls for temporary protective strategies.

Suicide is extremely rare in mothers with babies and young children, but in those with a severe PND (for example during puerperal psychosis, a manic state, psychotic depression and, less so, melancholic depression) the risk is up to 80 times higher in the first year with a young baby. The risk is still low: 1–2 per 1000 mothers, but highest in the first month. Desperation that can lead to suicide is most commonly a result of the woman developing nihilistic preoccupations that she—and sometimes the baby too—has no future in such a bleak world and that ending it all is the 'only way out' and the only way to achieve 'relief from the pain'.

Such distressing states are extremely rare and almost invariably respond completely to treatment. They are regarded as psychiatric emergencies as the mother and her baby need to be protected. On recovery, some mothers will have no memory of this time. Many do, however, as the two descriptions below attest. Note particularly Francesca and Pam's passionate reassurance of recovery to mothers who are experiencing a PND that threatens to crush them.

Francesca sets the scene:

Survivor

I am a survivor. I say that with my whole heart. There was a time in my life when I did not believe I would ever feel or smile again, a time when the ache in my heart was so bad I was prepared to take my own life to make the pain stop, though it was not really what I wanted to do. If not for the support of my family and a few really good friends I would not be here to write this today.

I had just given birth to our beautiful daughter: a long-awaited miracle for us. It was a horrendous birth with a lot of complications, but when she was first born it was the most joyous and happy time of our life. Two weeks later all began to change. I was readmitted to hospital and required urgent surgery. I awoke feeling flat, teary and incompetent—unable to move and unable to care for my beautiful child. I had no appetite and just wanted to sleep. Feelings of hopelessness seeped through me. I was allowed to go home from hospital four days later. The feelings remained but I just brushed them under the carpet, trying to remain strong, pushing through and telling myself this was meant to be the best time of my life.

I had been home for 48 hours when it hit. That is the only way to describe the onset. For some people it gradually creeps up and they often don't get diagnosed for months. For me it was like a wall crashing onto me. People ask how I knew I had depression. Well, I couldn't miss it. I was a mess, lying in the foetal position on my bed, rocking back and forth, not wanting to be left alone, crying out in emotional agony, unable to move, wanting someone to take my daughter away as I was not good enough for her. Luckily my husband was home and quickly rang my parents and the doctor. Within four hours I was readmitted to hospital, sedated, a 24-hour nurse with me and an order of detainment issued.

I spent a week in that hospital, sedated to calm me to a functioning point. My daughter stayed with me and I was encouraged to take care of her, although I did have a nurse sit at my door continually. I was reminded by my sister later that the nurse had to sit outside my door as the scratch of her pen writing on the paper drove me to distraction, as did her turning the pages of the book she was reading. To hear that now is incomprehensible—that someone can be so mentally unwell—and that that person was me. I was transferred to a psychiatric hospital that had a mother-and-baby unit—the worst day of my life, being driven through the gates of this hospital that only the crazies went to. I did not want to stay but I knew I couldn't go home.

In some ways I was blessed. My postnatal depression did not affect the way I felt about my daughter. I truly loved her and wanted the world for her; I just wanted her to have a new mother—someone who could take care of her, someone who would not let her down. At this point I was even too scared to pick her up as I was afraid I would drop her.

I remained in this hospital for eight weeks. My poor husband and parents. This was our first child and their first grandchild. My husband went back to work on the recommendation of the doctors, so every day he would visit after work until about 11 pm and then he would go home. My parents also visited every day when my husband was at work and cooked and brought in meals for us.

I had never been on antidepressants before so there was a lot of trial and error. That was my main reason to remain in hospital, and also to re-educate me to increase my confidence and self-worth about being a mother. I met a truly amazing friend there with whom I still have contact today. We understood each other and what we were going through. I lost a lot of people who I thought were friends. They couldn't cope or chose not to cope and didn't understand what I was experiencing. I understand that—prior to this happening to me, I didn't understand depression: I also thought, 'Just get over it.' How wrong I was. It still hurts, though, when I had had those friends for years and have never heard from them since.

When I finally came home I had been in hospital for three months in total with only two days at home during that period. It was a major adjustment for me. Initially my wonderful parents came and sat with me, from the minute my husband left for work until he came home. I took care of my daughter the whole time but just needed their company to cope and not be alone. I felt so alone. The pain and hurt in my heart was still there—an empty ache that would not go away. I wanted it to stop and on a few occasions my dad had to hold me down and take my car keys away. I truly couldn't see a way through the pain and never believed I could be well or feel happiness again. But I did.

I began to try everything possible to overcome these feelings. I commenced walking every day for at least an hour and a half, my poor old dad or husband in tow helping me with the pusher. I started to read, a lot. I would read books on positive affirmations and put sayings on my walls, fridge, anywhere. It was during this time I began to take more responsibility—I had to push through this for my family, not just me. One day whilst walking I laughed. I mean I really laughed, and a little hope shone through.

It has been a long road travelled, a struggle, a curse and a blessing. People ask me, 'How has it been a blessing?' It is a blessing as I have changed. I have turned my life around. I took a negative and turned it into a positive. It is a blessing as I now live life. I see things happening around me, and people and nature and emotions. Work is no longer my definer, I am no longer an over-achiever. I enjoy the moment, the here and now. I have learned to appreciate what I have rather than always wanting more. I now appreciate me for who I am as an individual. I am not consumed anymore by what others think and I hope that I am empowering my daughter with the same skills, which I never would have learned if not for my postnatal depression.

I have recently come off all my medication with the help of my psychiatrist, but if I have to go back on . . . that is okay too. If I had a heart problem I wouldn't hesitate to be on medication so why should depression be any different? I tell others what I have been through and hold my head high. If I can help just one other mother to realise she needs help and that things will become okay, I have done my job.

Our daughter is now 6 years old and I never believed I would say this, but we are trying for another child. I am scared stiff to be honest but I also know we can get through it. All the struggles and triumphs are definitely worth the risk.

I am a survivor.

A tragedy averted

Pam also tells a heart-rending story whose ending could have been very different. She felt that she was 'drowning in emptiness' when she set out from home one day to end the pain that she felt she could not endure for another minute. She tells the events of that afternoon:

I tucked them into bed for their afternoon nap. My 5-month-old in her cot, asleep for now (she did not sleep much at all, night or day) and my 2-year-old in his bed. This was my time. I went back in to my son and kissed him goodbye, told him I loved him and was very sorry but I knew (well, that's what I truly believed in that state) that I was doing the best thing for everyone.

We were living with my parents at the time, as was my sister, her husband and their 7-month-old daughter. I was meant to be dropping off coathangers to my mother-in-law who was helping me with some ironing. So I collected them and said I was heading off. I said goodbye to my sister and kissed my niece, who was like another daughter to me. She was sitting in her highchair having a snack; she looked me in the eye then let out a horrific scream. I was a little rattled and my sister could not understand why she would scream at me like that. I knew she had seen something in me that day that was not right. I left anyway. I knew what I had to do.

I drove the ten minutes to my mother-in-law's then kept driving right past her house to the top of the mountain. I knew there was an area where a car could fit through. I could not see any other way out.

I contemplated for a long time whether to call my husband or not; he was at work and had no idea where this day had led me. Not that I had any idea either what was in store for me. I finally decided that I owed it to him to let him know. I just wanted to tell him—I did not want him to talk me out of it. Nothing could help me anymore. I had to end this pain . . . I could not take it for another minute.

I pulled the car over to the side of the road and rang him. I can only imagine what he went through in that phone call. The sheer panic in his voice did not register to me at the time. I was so numb and could not feel anything anymore. I tried to just tell him what I was going to do and that I needed to tell him how much I loved him and our children and to please forgive me.

Somehow in that phone call my husband convinced me to drive straight to him at work. I cannot remember the 20-minute drive; I have no idea how I made it there but thank God I did. He is my angel and I owe him my life. He saved me from this horrible disease and from myself. He saved our family and he was my rock.

He took me straight to my childhood GP who saw me immediately and put me on antidepressants on the spot. The only reason I was not admitted to hospital was that we were living at my parents' house, but I was not allowed to be left alone. There I began my slow recovery.

I had considered suicide before but had never talked about it to anyone nor had I tried to carry it out. I remember locking the bathroom door on many occasions and taking a long bath. I would put my head under the water for as long as I could, wondering if it was possible to drown yourself. Under there it was peaceful; it felt like I could escape the pain. It would feel sometimes in the depth of my depression that there was physical pain. I felt so heavy in my chest sometimes that I wished I could just sink into the ground and be swallowed up.

There must have been many warnings around me but it was so hard for loved ones to know the true extent of my emotions because I found that even though I could cry all day sometimes and be visibly upset, the depression made me shut down in so many other ways. It was a very lonely battle. I believe making everyone understand why you are feeling the way you are before you have a label to put on it is extremely hard. It's hard to verbalise what's happening to you when you're in that state. Once I was diagnosed with PND it was easier to tell people why I was feeling the way I was. I could just tell them I had postnatal depression and that was all I had to say.

Unfortunately, I did not recognise I needed help until I was at breaking point. What I would wish for anyone who has the bad luck to have this disease is to have it recognised early. No one should have to go through what my family and I went through. Education is the key to catching it early—and not just educating the mothers-to-be, but everyone around them, because I was not able to recognise what was happening to me. There was always a reason in my mind, like 'when she starts to sleep' or 'when the colic ends' or 'when the crying stops' I will feel better.

What helped me? Medication was a given: I needed it and there was no denying that and it worked. The other main thing was support, and that came in many forms. First and foremost was my husband. I truly don't believe I would be here today if it was not for him. And I don't know how anyone would get through PND without a supportive, loving, patient and non-judgemental partner.

Other support that I needed was a good GP. I say 'good' because I don't think every doctor out there is good with PND and sometimes shopping around and paying for what you get can make a world of difference. I believe that having a good GP in place before pregnancy *is extremely important for recognising emotional changes in you. This would have been very helpful for me during my first pregnancy, as I suffered mood swings and inability to cope during periods of this pregnancy but I did not realise that it was even possible to have depression during pregnancy. I also realised after this first child was 9 months old that I felt like a cloud had lifted off me. I definitely had PND with him but did not recognise it until after it went away on its own.*

Family and close friends were also extremely helpful. When your partner is at work of a day it's good to know that someone else has your back. I had two close friends who would call or visit me each day. I know this must have been a burden of sorts for them but it was so important to my recovery. As I was living with my immediate family they were also a very big support. Sometimes I think the generation gap with my mother and her old perception of depression made it hard on me. Even though she would not admit it, I felt she was ashamed of the fact that I was 'not coping' as she would say. As a mother with PND you feel like you have somehow failed and you put shame on yourself—you don't need anyone else doing this as well.

Along with regular visits to my GP, I attended weekly counselling sessions for a time. These were helpful, although I wish there were more support groups available. I wish there was group counselling available where I could have spoken with other mothers going through the same experiences. As the other mothers around me were not suffering from PND, it was often very lonely.

The year this happened to me was 2004, so I have come a long way since then; it feels like a lifetime ago. I have gone on to have another baby and am very pleased to say I did not suffer postnatal depression again. I did, however, have everyone on standby and on the lookout for it, including doctors, family and friends. It was a big decision to have baby number three after what I had gone through.

Pam now has a contented and busy family life, despite such a terrifying episode. We use her words to convey the gift of hope: 'Education, preparation, support and talking about it are the keys to conquering

PND.' She voices a common theme—that if her story helps just one person, then it is worth broadcasting.

Her message: 'Please look for and accept help. Understand that you're not alone and that you *will* recover.'

nine

Tackling stigma and mothers' guilt

The joys of parents are secret, and so are their griefs and fears.

Francis Bacon[1]

Mental illness has long been stigmatised and, while the last decade has seen distinct improvement, there is still a heavy stigma attached to the perinatal disorders.

In his book *A First-rate Madness*, psychiatrist Nassir Ghaemi considers that prejudice against mental illness crosses all societies and all historical epochs. He thinks that intuitive responses and beliefs have grown out of this prejudice over millennia and they will not change easily or soon. Nonetheless, he wrote, 'the indisputable fact remains that the border between health and illness is porous. Some aspects of mental health are found in even the most severe mental illness, and some aspects of mental illness reside in the most mentally healthy person. Abnormal, illogical thought processes are common in normal, mentally healthy people.'[2]

WHY DO WE STIGMATISE THOSE WHO ARE DIFFERENT?

The origins of stigmatisation probably have evolutionary importance, driven by innate survival mechanisms that cause us to scan the environment and draw back from anything atypical. In essence, stigma operates to divide a population into 'us' and 'not us', but in reality we're all part of the same group.

Where is the boundary between normal and abnormal? How can we narrow this distance? The medium is empathy. While stigmatising and judgemental responses may have some biological underpinnings, they are socially irrational. If stigma becomes entrenched it leads to the stereotyping and prejudices that endlessly drive one culture or race to suppress another. In this context, a mother with a mood disorder denies her distress, puts on a brave face and resists declaring her inner turmoil. Thus she avoids being judged, blamed and seen as a failed and atypical mother. But at what cost?

Psychologist Gordon Allport, in his book *The Nature of Prejudice*, stated that while it took years of labour and billions of dollars to uncover the secret of the atom, it would take a greater investment to gain the secrets of 'man's irrational nature'[3]—that it is easier to smash an atom than a prejudice. In some ways he is right. The smashing of the atom was work undertaken by only a fraction of society; the challenge of redressing prejudices, in contrast, needs to be tackled by every member of a community. Australian culture is moving in this direction—challenging prejudices based on race, religion, gender, sexual orientation and age—but redressing each stigma requires a campaign and strategies, and a community prepared to change its mindset. There is, at least, an awareness of such issues and a greater weighting to egalitarian values.

HOW DO WE FIGHT STIGMA?

A key strategy of destigmatisation and increasing social inclusion is to put a human face to the issue. If we can, or are made to, put ourselves in the position of the victim, the oppressed, the stigmatised, then our prejudices can be dissolved by empathy—the capacity for each of us to project ourselves into the life of another person and better understand their differences and difficulties.

Empathy is not sympathy. Empathy is not hierarchical; it is based on equality. It comes from trying to understand how the other person feels. Empathy underlies the accounts in this book. The wish to promote understanding and reconcile the views of the observer with those of the sufferer was a common driver for these mothers, our everyday heroines, to broadcast their stories and to firmly defy any feelings of exposure, self-blame and shame. We hope that entry into the distressed and distressing world of these women with perinatal depression—intrinsically caring and decent people bearing the scars and lessons of their mood disorder—will advance destigmatisation.

Self-stigmatisation is a barrier to admitting difficulties

Accepting help was by far the biggest stumbling block for Ellie. Social stigma was a big hindrance to recovery and it is only now that she can empathise with—and truly comprehend—the emotional nightmare of admitting to a mood disorder.

She believed that no one could—or for that matter wanted to—look behind her facade. They were fooled by the competence she portrayed. She knew that *something* was wrong. She struggled on alone for months and finally diagnosed herself from a list of symptoms in a parenting book. However, recognition was still another world from acceptance. There were answers but they were not the answers she wanted:

Motherhood is supposed to be a time of joy, elation and the beautiful expression of new life. Indeed, after the birth of my first child I would have agreed—I didn't even experience the baby blues.

But after the birth of my second child, well, there didn't seem to be that much joy around. I was overdue, had a difficult labour with an epidural that didn't work, post-birth haemorrhaging and a 10-pound [4.5-kilogram] baby who lost weight rapidly due to severe dietary allergies. Any and all could have added up to postnatal depression. Because frankly, after my daughter was born, my mind became a murky place to inhabit. I did not bond well with my new baby and life got on top of me.

I knew I had to get answers somehow. I had no desire to continue this half-life with its unpredictable mood swings and irrational reactions. I wanted escape from the restlessness and dissatisfaction, the anxiety attacks and their consequences: domestic problems, low self-esteem and raw irritability.

When I finally found the reason for the way I was feeling, well, telling other people—that was too hard. Admitting that depression, a mood disorder, had stopped me, had almost defeated me. No. I was not ready to admit to that. I was, and am still, too proud for that. I did not want to be labelled throughout the remainder of my life as depressed, to see the pity in another's eyes and actions.

Would I rather carry this burden alone? Absolutely!

Ultimately, of course, I couldn't. And it came time to tell my husband that I thought I had postnatal depression. But even then I was unable physically to utter those simple words: 'I have depression.' Instead, I opened the book and made him read the section on postnatal depression. Then we set about getting around this obstacle.

Rani wrote that even though we have come so far in confronting the stigma around PND a pulse of judgement still silently pumps through our veins:

Celebs lose their baby weight and are back at work within weeks, and mothers are trying to emulate them. I believe that the media should take a lot of the blame for fanning the flame of unrealistic perceptions, which then fuel 'ordinary' mothers to expect that from each other.

The Mummy Wars breed mistrust: fears about being vulnerable, strictures about being open and speaking from your heart. This fast-paced and mechanised world has little time for frank connection. Mothers' groups are fantastic, but there is still a clique culture there too.

I believe there needs to be a return to real women's circles so we can heal, and reveal ourselves as mothers and women in an absolute absence of judgement.

Grace also articulated the belief that while the stigma attached to mental illness is appalling in itself, the stigma attached to PND is worse still. She observed that already these mothers are vulnerable and feel as if they've failed some 'ancient initiation into the secret joys of motherhood'. She also noted that as they lug around their feelings of guilt, shame, failure and a whole lot of other burdensome emotions, society puts another pressure on them—its fear that they'll harm their child:

> *I know this might sound a little bitter but I think it's time to expose a lot of the myths surrounding postnatal depression. I don't know how many websites I visited that kept pressing the view that I might harm my baby: even the hospital's counsellor asked about whether I had thoughts of harming my child. Not surprisingly, this so-called assistance made me feel worse.*
>
> *Often, it is the fear of this itself that drives the illness in the first place. Am I good enough? What if I hurt the child—pull too hard, can't support her properly, drop her accidentally, trip down some stairs? What if she eats something and chokes? Or has an allergy? Or vomits in her sleep? What if she rolls over in bed and can't breathe properly? It was not the fear of hurting my little girl deliberately but the fear of being incompetent and forgetting something important that might put her at risk. Admittedly, many of these fears were irrational and required therapy to help me counter them with positive thoughts. But it was hard, really hard. Sleep deprivation blurs the line between the rational and irrational so it is difficult to tell where the logic lies. It was never about 'not having an emotional connection' or the risk of harming her. I have always loved my daughter unreservedly—that is the whole point.*
>
> *No wonder women don't readily put their hand up and ask for help when they're struggling. They probably feel the same fears I did when I presented myself to the hospital counsellor: 'Why am I in this situation? I must be incompetent. This is evidence that I'm losing my mind. Are they going to take my baby from me?' None of this happened and I was given valuable help and, ultimately, skills that have stayed with me, but you are so vulnerable when you are ill like that and you don't know where a plea for help will take you.*

HAVE I BROKEN THE BABY?

It is believed that at the baby's birth a 'guilt chip' is inserted into every mother.

Anon.

In the 1950s, the American psychiatrist Jules Masserman published an article arguing that we hold three 'normal' delusions,[4] one being that our mother loves us without reservation. This fits with our idealised view of mothering—as a font of ever-giving unconditional love, a source of never-ending emotional nurturance. This societal belief acts as a particularly potent driver of self-stigmatisation in any woman experiencing PND. As depression has eroded her capacity to love and give care to her baby for some period of time, the mother considers with dismay whether her emotional unavailability has damaged her baby psychologically and perhaps permanently. This concern is so guilt-inducing, so much the antithesis of being a 'good mother', that it is rarely voiced by women during their depressive episode or for decades after, and sometimes never. This uncertainty fuels guilt and shame.

We have attended support groups for mothers who had been referred for—or had sought—assistance in managing their depression. Some of these plucky women had embarked on motherhood while managing their pre-existing mood disorder and were finding the juggling difficult. Others had experienced a heightening of some predisposing personality traits—such as anxiousness or perfectionism—together with a partner who was having his own problems. Still others had been floored by their little one's physical and possible intellectual disabilities, or a multiple birth.

We asked members of two groups 'How are you able to relate to your baby when you're having difficulties yourself?' but refrained from asking this of any other groups out of a sense that the question was intrusive, distressing and painful. Each time the question was met with an uncomfortable silence, in stark contrast to the eager, generous and frank exchanges in response to other questions. One mother became teary, noting that her depression had not been detected until her little girl was 9 months old. During the hour of the session, however, her child was curious, engaged and responsive, trundling around, exploring and then returning to her mother's lap. Her mother was convinced, though, that her period of depression had damaged her baby.

Mother–child attachment and bonding

There has been much research into mother–child attachment and bonding, and we are now aware of how finely attuned a baby is to its mother. We also know that distinct lack of parental care can contribute to a child's low self-esteem and increase their chance of depression. But there is no evidence from this research that a mother's depression can leave a permanent negative imprint on her child. Neglect has to be gross and cruel, and indifference callous for it to have any effect. While this is reassuring, it also has elements of 'It all depends'.

Several studies report that, while PND predicted lower self-care in the mother and poorer levels of household and personal functioning, no difference was found in the actual care of her infant (regardless of the baby's gender or wakefulness or the parental income), indicating that a woman can manage to provide good physical care for her baby regardless of her depressive symptoms.[5] The mother may, because of her depression, mistakenly perceive deficits in her mothering skills that are neither as severe as she thinks nor as pervasive an influence on her infant.

Sydney GP Dr Vered Gordon adds:

The way I look at it is if the mother had been injured in a car accident or had a cardiac event or was diagnosed with MS when her baby was little—yes, there would be a separation or an attachment disruption, but no one would feel guilty or ashamed, it would be accepted as part of what life brings. The focus would be on getting the mother well ASAP and repairing any damage to the attachment between mother and baby as soon as feasible. It is another aspect of stigmatisation of mental illness that women feel (and are made to feel) responsible for the illness and the impact of the illness as though they could have chosen not to be ill.

Dr Gordon says of the memories of now-adult children about a mother with untreated depression:

Some of my patients do remember their depressed mothers but this is usually in the context of a mother who never sought help. They feel hurt and angry that their parent never tried to do something about their depression, despite the burden it placed on them as children. Clearly this is a very different scenario from that of the mother of a young infant who identifies her depression, seeks treatment, is returned to health and is then quickly able to restore the secure mother–child attachment bond.

The effect of parental depression

Research indicates that there can be long-term effects on the cognitive, behavioural and emotional development of children whose mothers had *significant* and severe PND. Possible consequences are most evident with mothers whose PND was severe and chronic (long-term) and who did not effectively access help. Untreated depression lingers and fluctuates, making it difficult for a mother to interact positively and sensitively with her child, depleting her energy to play, sing and read with the child. Her symptoms dissipate and recur, making her parenting less consistent. And when a mother cannot respond to her child, the child tends not to respond so well to her.

An American study into the causes of PND[6] observed that ongoing depression was more likely in mothers from a disadvantaged background with low educational levels and high rates of unemployment. Even in this challenging setting the researchers used a brief treatment intervention that helped mothers to identify stigmas, practise relaxation techniques, reduce negative thinking, and link maternal mood and behaviour with child mood and behaviour. This helped reduce their symptoms of depression and improved their perspective on their child's behaviour. Children (aged 4 and younger) whose mothers received the therapy also showed fewer behavioural problems.

Neutralising disruption to the mother–baby bond

While the mother is recovering from PND, the baby can draw on other people as attachment figures. Such people will often come forward spontaneously but, if not, the mother should not hesitate to seek the assistance of family and friends in enriching the baby's emotional environment.

Quality of other parenting figures

The death of a parent is traumatic and emotionally perturbing for a child but, if the remaining parent and other 'parent figures' (such as the grandmother, brother or aunt) are supportive over subsequent years, there is no evidence of any permanent substantive effect. Separation of parents is also generally traumatic for the child at the time but again, subject to the key parent (and any other parent figures) being supportive and caring of the child, there is no permanent substantial impact.

Quality of subsequent intimate relationships

A study of women who had experienced traumatic childhoods and been placed in girls' homes[7] found that those who subsequently formed a relationship with an uncaring or abusive partner were highly likely to be depressed in adulthood, while those who chose a caring partner were no more likely to be depressed than women in the general community. So, while earlier uncaring parenting set up a predisposition for the offspring to low self-esteem and depression, that susceptibility was reduced or averted by establishing a caring relationship.

An earlier study found that women whose mother had died early in their life could neutralise this risk factor for depression by accessing care from their remaining parent or, as an adult, selected a caring partner.[8]

So while early parent–child bond disruptions can be very distressing, negative effects are not necessarily permanent. While PND can disrupt the mother–child bond, such effects can be averted by the support of other parent figures (partner, family and friends), and by treatment for the mother's depression. Children have a self-correcting capacity and can bounce back from earlier distressing experiences— subject to their care being 'good enough'. All of this argues against a mother's PND having any substantial lasting effect on their child.

DITCH THE CAPE: TREAT MISTAKES AS OPPORTUNITIES TO LEARN

We hope that, as a new mother, you will not assume that you have to be Superwoman (beware the kryptonite!). The change from 'just the two of us' into your own blend of family is a learning curve. Its shape is tailored by and is unique to you. There is no standard mother, no commandments, and no benchmark baby. You're the only mother your baby has had. The baby isn't any the wiser that you forgot to bathe them for the first week. They're not responsive to opinion polls, and are complete pragmatists in their own little way. They haven't read the books, either. The best advice when you make a mistake is to learn from it: as one mum says, 'that way your kids can see firsthand how to deal with getting things wrong'. Apologise, forget it and move on.

One aspect of parenting is not perhaps apparent before you actually have children. It is their continuing legacy. Your heart is in trust to another in a way that is very different from previous experiences of the boyfriend–girlfriend variety. The authors of the book *Sh*tty Mum: The Parenting Guide for the Rest of Us* warn of this vulnerability when they observe that you may feel that as a parent 'you are always one dumb mistake away from unfathomable grief'.[9] Though all parents are savvy about the lack of sleep and endless expenses, 'the worst part is that, for the rest of your life, your heart can be broken'. They warn about the tendency to become emotionally shredded by every family tragedy you read about or hear on the news. They advise that you can't 'replay each well-publicized crime or accident as if it had happened to your family' or else you couldn't function. Skip the 'What if [*insert unthinkable tragedy*] . . .?' question and concentrate on your own here and now.

Deliver yourself from judgement

> *The good enough mother is one who gives her child what it needs to grow up. The good enough child is one who manages to grow up, and in doing so, is able to recognise her mother's humanity.*
>
> Emily Wilson[10]

'What kind of mother would . . .?' Columnist and author Erma Bombeck mused that this familiar phrase is 'conceived in innocence, carried with pomposity, delivered with vehemence and born of condemnation'.[11] And it is often only after you become a mother that such judgement, hopefully, turns to compassion. She says, 'Let none of you judge mothers until you have walked in their feet of clay.' Grace, an essayist, makes this appeal: 'please remember you're the *only* mother your baby knows or wants. You have their best interests at heart and know them the best in the world. You can't damage your baby with momentary lapses.'

It seems counterintuitive, but we suspect that an episode of PND may actually improve or add a deeper quality to the mother–child bond. A study of people attending the Black Dog Institute Depression Clinic for management of their mood disorder asked them whether they felt that having a mood disorder had any advantages.[12] Sixty-two per cent of those diagnosed with bipolar disorder and nearly one-quarter of those diagnosed with depression named some positives, particularly greater empathy, increased self-awareness, and enhanced relationships with family and friends. Similarly, and as you will have already noted, the majority of our essayists describe how after overcoming their depression they appreciated their child more and had a deeper relationship with that child over the years. And they themselves were endowed with greater resilience, insight and compassion.

ten

Managing a mood disorder and maintaining recovery

Prenatal: When your life was still somewhat your own.

Anon.

We believe that a woman who has sought help for a perinatal mood disorder should be given a diagnosis and formulation, along with a level of confidence from the clinician (such as 'I'm certain this is the baby blues and that it will lift in a few days' or 'In light of your symptoms and family history, I'm fairly confident you have a melancholic depression'). As such conditions respond well to treatment and can be brought under control, the clinician can genuinely offer hope of an optimistic outcome. Most people respond positively, relieved to know what they have to deal with, seek targeted information, and are progressively able to separate their condition from their own identity. A diagnosis helps sufferers come out of the darkness. Others take longer to adjust and need additional help to come to terms with it.

TREATMENTS FOR DEPRESSION DURING PREGNANCY AND AFTER THE BIRTH

As we have seen, the symptoms of mood disorders and anxiety that occur amongst women of childbearing age are similar to those that occur at other times of life. The treatment choices may differ, however, to avoid damage to the foetus during pregnancy and the infant during breastfeeding. Options include counselling, psychological therapies and medications.

The types of treatments and how they are prioritised vary according to the nature, severity and subtype of the disorder. Psychological therapies and counselling are appropriate and sufficient for many women—especially those with non-melancholic subtypes of depression (see Chapter 1) in which stresses from life events, relationship disturbances or personality patterns contribute to the difficulties of coping with a newborn baby.

For melancholic and psychotic depression, bipolar disorder and puerperal psychosis (see Chapter 1), medication is generally the first-line treatment (see the Appendix for the safety of differing medications during pregnancy and breastfeeding). Advisory centres such as MotherSafe[1] provide up-to-date information to women during this time, with consultations available by phone or in person. Doctors avoid the use of medication that might affect the developing foetus or the breastfeeding infant but if the mother is gravely ill and disabled, they will reach a compromise between the benefits and disadvantages.

ECT may also be used to treat severe episodes (such as agitated melancholia and puerperal psychosis; see Chapter 1), as it allows for quick recovery and so minimal disruption to the mother–baby relationship.

Strategies to keep mood disorders at bay

During a depressive episode many strategies can help relieve depression and anxiety and distract from stress. These include exercise, yoga, meditation, repeating mantras, learning to recognise and accept emotions and understanding their context, maintaining a healthy diet (we recommend daily fish oil supplement), achieving enough sleep (an essential, not a luxury), and getting involved in supportive mothers' groups and playgroups. All social support is beneficial (but of course avoid people who bring you down or are constantly critical). Exercise is also very helpful—some places offer exercise programs tailored for new mothers (such as Pramercise) but even working out to a DVD or on a games console at home makes a difference.

Prioritising activities and juggling responsibilities is hard. Your mental health and resilience will be bolstered by allocating time for you to engage in activities for *yourself*. Your partner and family are in a position to encourage you to give yourself permission to put off things that don't really need to be done and to make use of support and friends. If they offer to do practical things, let them. A helpful question to ask yourself is, 'What would I do for my friend if I saw she was depressed?' Allow them to do the same for you. Time with your partner is also essential, so accept offers from trusted friends to babysit. A quiet dinner or a movie allows you to remember that you are not only mother but woman and partner as well.

The simplest treatments are those that are supportive, educational, and give you and your partner some understanding and acceptance of the causes of your particular condition and strategies for coping. Some days you may feel as if you've slipped back again. See it for the temporary setback it is. Depression can sometimes be triggered by unnecessary worrying, lack of information and incorrect beliefs about a situation, so correct information will help allay your concerns and confer a sense of control. Doctors, midwives, child and family health nurses, and parent educators all play a part in providing information about pregnancy and the behaviours of newborns. They can also correct misinformation. It's so important to ask questions rather than worry in silence. If your depressive or anxiety symptoms persist in spite of reassuring information and support, you should consider other treatment approaches. Ask for these if they're not automatically provided.

Psychotherapy or counselling

Proven psychotherapeutic approaches include cognitive behaviour therapy (CBT) and interpersonal therapy (IPT), both of which teach the necessary skills to identify and deal with situations that trigger or increase distress. CBT assumes that much of the sufferer's distress comes from the way they see the world, view themselves and anticipate their future. We each have an 'attributional' system, and CBT aims to teach us to recognise and modify views that could lead to depression. CBT also seeks to modify behaviours, such as encouraging a shy person to be more assertive. IPT focuses on strategies for dealing with current stressors, particularly those to do with relating to other people.

These therapies can be undertaken individually or in groups, and weekly sessions are generally recommended. The first six to ten sessions may be subsidised if your GP draws up a qualifying mental health plan. As well as psychologists, some counsellors, social workers, midwives and nurses also have experience with these techniques.

Women who have longstanding problems arising from their childhood may find other forms and lengthier psychotherapies beneficial. Couples' counselling can be useful for problems in the parents' relationship, while some therapists will work with the mother and baby together or with both parents together in assisting a mother with PND.

Practical strategies

A mother with PND is both depressed and stressed. This is a time when her relationship with her own mother or mother-in-law comes into its own. Hopefully their relationship is one of sufficient trust and support, and is positive and uncritical. The new mother needs her stress levels reduced and she needs to sleep. The father, too, is still adapting to his new role in their family and could do with some relief.

A new mother must take some time for herself to recharge her batteries so she has the energy to look after those in her care. She must be given, and give herself, permission to be kinder to herself.

In particular, consider these four ideas:

1. Break your day into segments, and maintain some markers of its progress (a morning walk, morning tea, a nap if the baby goes to sleep).
2. Concentrate on the current section of the day, focusing on what to do now.
3. Note each thing accomplished, no matter how slight it might seem. Set modest expectations rather than 'mission impossible' goals.

4. Do at least one 'want to do' activity (see table below) in each time segment.

A prescription for good health

Adapt the details of this timetable to suit your routine, but follow it daily.

	Need to do (non-negotiable)	Could do (or skip)	Want to do
Early morning	Get dressed (put clothes out the night before) Feed and change baby Put baby to bed Put on a load of washing Have something to eat	Fold nappies and clothes Make bed (pull up doona)	Walk around block while partner minds baby before going to work Give partner washing to drop off at a laundromat Sit down, have a coffee and look at a mummy blog for advice or amusement
Mid-morning	Put out washing Feed and change baby Play with then settle baby Make lunch	Clean one room of its more obvious mess Vacuum Shop for groceries or order them online for delivery	Go for walk in the park with baby Read a magazine
Early afternoon	Feed and change baby Put baby to bed Eat lunch	Clean up kitchen Ask your mum to iron some essentials	Have a nap Catch up with a friend Go out and have a coffee (perhaps your mum can do a short babysit)
Later afternoon	Feed and change baby Put baby into bouncinette Tidy up enough to be able to find stuff Bring in washing Eat a snack	Fold washing Prepare (or unfreeze) dinner	Ask partner to bring home dinner Discuss day with partner Watch television Relax in bath

FOUR STORIES OF SEVERE POSTNATAL CONDITIONS AND WHAT HELPED

Carlita's story, 'You can't always tell by looking', describes how she was confounded and silenced by the many people who said to her, 'You don't look depressed', 'You don't seem the type' and 'What have you got to be depressed about?' As she observed, if only those factors had granted her immunity from PND! What these basically well-meaning people couldn't see from the outside looking in were her family history, biological make-up, life events, stressful circumstances and lack of support:

Indeed, to the outside world I'm healthy, happily married, have two gorgeous children, live in a nice suburb, am well educated and work part-time in the legal profession. But if you scratch beneath the surface you learn about risk factors and vulnerability and, with the benefit of hindsight, I might have considered my own mental health in a little more depth prior to giving birth rather than dismissing the small segment on depression in prenatal classes as irrelevant.

Well, you live and learn. I am well placed to provide an insight into the condition, both from the perspective of a first-time mother experiencing her first major episode of postnatal depression, and from the perspective of managing the condition throughout a further pregnancy and first year after birth. And I'm not alone. In fact, the more people I am open with about my experience the more people share their stories with me. I never cease to be surprised—but I shouldn't be—postnatal depression is the number one complication of pregnancy.

Close your eyes and imagine you are on a plane that is about to crash. At the same time you have just been told that your dearest relative has died. Your physical and emotional states would be in overdrive and meltdown at the same time. Well, that is how depression and anxiety felt for me. To say that it was the most debilitating and enduring form of suffering I have ever experienced would be an understatement.

I felt intense love for my daughter from the moment she was born. She was planned, healthy and much loved. I had a natural, drug-free birth and no major problems with breastfeeding.

But I worried.

She cried a lot and was difficult to soothe. She didn't respond to physical touch and, after a frantic call to Karitane at 3 am, we started pushing her vigorously in her pram to get her to sleep. I had some discomfort following the birth and became anxious about it. I was also scared that I might get mastitis. Sleep deprivation kicked in. My husband and I were novices when it came to looking after babies. We received a lot of conflicting advice. My mother was not available for practical or emotional support, I have no siblings and my in-laws lived some distance away. Our little girl got sick with a chest infection and we had to go to hospital. Then I got sick with a cough.

These issues by themselves were nothing extraordinary but, in combination with other risk factors, spelt trouble. These included:

- *a family history on the maternal side of depression, anxiety and bipolar disorder*
- *a very distressing miscarriage two years earlier with ongoing consequences requiring specialist treatment with hormones for a year*
- *the death of my father in an accident when I was tiny and the subsequent grief*
- *a complicated relationship with a mother who has suffered long-term mental illness herself*
- *a series of stressful events during my pregnancy, including the still-birth of a friend's baby, and witnessing a serious car accident*
- *the death of my best friend's father shortly after our daughter was born*
- *a history of hormonal sensitivity and PMT with insomnia and mood swings*
- *unstable living arrangements*
- *a legal job involving working with people in extreme crises*
- *an analytical mind, a need for control and a tendency to ruminate*
- *a long-term history of unrecognised and untreated anxiety, social anxiety and obsessive tendencies*
- *a husband with a long-term untreated mood disorder (but very supportive otherwise).*

Hmmm!

I actually thought I was coping well and even waxed lyrical to a friend about the joys of having a baby—and then I crashed. I developed acute insomnia; acute anxiety (about my inability to sleep, our daughter's sleep, my own health, our daughter's health, fear of being alone); obsessive looping thoughts that bombarded me constantly ('I'm going to die', 'I'm going to be sick forever', 'I'm going to Hell', 'I'm going to be separated from my baby'); religious ruminations and ruminations about the death of my father and my relationship with my mother (funny how you really think about the parenting you've received when you become a parent yourself); crying—a lot; chronic exhaustion; aches and pains; sensitivity to pain and noise; outbursts of irritability (out of character for someone who once won an office party award for 'never spitting the dummy'); normal emotions magnified a thousand times, with no control over them; loss of libido; self-loathing; feeling completely overwhelmed; thinking people were judging me; raving on and on about my condition and being unable to stop; guilt over anything and everything; loss of interest in anything; crap concentration and thinking everything was too hard (I couldn't even read or watch television); feeling incapable of looking after our daughter; difficulty making decisions; feeling estranged from our daughter and at other times overly focused on her; feeling that I couldn't go on.

Ugh!

And Ugh!

What helped

- *The enduring love and loyalty of my husband*
- *My own persevering nature*
- *Calling out for help, and taking responsibility for my treatment*
- *Hospitalisation, medication trial and error, a good psychiatrist and psychologist, cognitive behavioural therapy*
- *Practical and emotional support from family and friends, including church members who listened to me, texted me during crises, cooked meals, cared for our daughter or took me to the doctors*
- *Getting out of the house with the baby, meeting other people and calling on community resources*

- *Exercise and relaxation strategies*
- *Drawing up lists of achievable goals and easy meals or activities with the baby*
- *Consciously appreciating simple activities—showers, cups of tea, a nice meal*
- *Joining a group of mothers who also welcomed extra support*
- *Learning how to achieve better balance, via websites and forums*
- *Limiting late nights and alcohol consumption, eating well, adding vitamin supplements*
- *Having a routine to the day with achievable targets*
- *Returning to work part-time and regaining an identity outside of being a mother.*

What didn't help

- *Being put in a room opposite the baby nursery while still exhausted after giving birth, and hearing babies cry all night*
- *The nurse who simply said 'lower your expectations' when I left the hospital for home and said nothing about depression*
- *The sleeping pills and beta blockers I was initially put on by my doctor*
- *My own mindset against depression and antidepressants—I resisted medication for a long time and wanted to breastfeed at all costs*
- *The medications that didn't work or gave me side effects*
- *The lack of support from my family about psychiatric treatment and a belief that Christians don't suffer from depression*
- *The ignorance of those who think they know about depression but don't or don't want to. I was once one of them.*

Fast forward six years

We now have a girl aged 6 and a boy aged 2. Following medication changes, relapses, a further miscarriage, a change of residence and advancing age (not to mention changing my mind a dozen or so times about whether we should risk it again for another baby), I confronted my greatest fear and we had a much-longed-for second child. I've found that it has been much easier parenting number two without the burden of severe PND.

*This time I remained on medications; saw my psychiatrist regu-
larly; saw a naturopath; organised to go into the mother-and-baby
unit immediately after birth for a few weeks; decided to breastfeed during the day and bottle-feed overnight so that I could sleep;
arranged for in-home care to help us overnight (free government
initiative—helped save my sanity); accepted all offers of help . . . such
as meal rosters and babysitting; and had much more confidence in
my parenting abilities and less guilt at not doing everything perfectly
or by myself.*

*I never assume now that people who look as though they are
coping are in fact coping.*

Annalese still finds it hard to talk about her experience with her
second baby. She was then a 28-year-old woman in a good marriage,
with a 3-year-old daughter and a 5-month-old baby boy. She had
enjoyed a busy corporate job. She saw herself as a high achiever and
very capable. She loved being a mother and had plenty of support.

Then one Saturday night:

*It was the only night my husband had been out in the previous
six months, and I was home alone. I remember feeling a bit tense
that day but I just put it down to lack of sleep. As my husband said
goodbye that night, on reflection, I felt that I had been getting more
anxious and uptight for some time. That night started as usual, my
newborn screaming and my 3-year-old being her lovely independent
self. I felt exhausted.*

*As I read a story to my daughter, baby screaming in the back-
ground, my whole body suddenly warmed up; it tingled all over and
sweat poured off me—yes, a panic attack. My heart was racing and
I was breathing heavily. I immediately ran out of the room, away
from the feeling that I might do something to hurt my daughter.
After calming down outside with some deep breathing and self-talk, I
managed to go back and read the rest of the story.*

*I wondered what on earth was happening to me, shocked and
terrified by the feeling I'd just had. This wasn't like me. What would
happen if I lost my mind? Could I do something impulsive? Were the*

kids in danger from me? My life would be over if something happened to them.

Thus the roller-coaster began.

Up until that Saturday night, I'd been telling myself to get on with things and that I just needed to get to three months and things would be better. I'd done the mother thing before and I'd coped well and enjoyed it. While I'd felt a little bit low at times with my first pregnancy, I was always able to carry on well enough.

Like a lot of mums, my expectations of myself are quite high and I'm used to being organised and in control. The problem was that I hadn't slept in about four months—stretching back before the birth. My baby boy was also a party animal, screaming day and night, and hardly off the boob or out of my arms. Add to that mix some significant family issues, some pre- and post-pregnancy health issues, unsuccessfully toilet training my older child and frequent doses of unhelpful advice—you could say that it was inevitable that something was going to give. My body and mind were at breaking point.

The next week was torture. My first step was to talk to my husband, although I was still hoping I could sleep it off and get back to feeling like me. After a visit to the early childhood centre I got an immediate spot in the local parent support centre, which offers day stays and counselling services. That helped a lot and I was hopeful I was going to get better. However, the following morning I still felt terrible and didn't want to be left alone with the kids or by myself. I was terrified that I'd had such thoughts about my kids, who I love so much. It then dawned on me that I might have PND, which I pretty much confirmed by doing the Edinburgh test on the beyond-blue website. I'd had this test after the birth of my baby boy but I'd felt fine at that time.

A GP appointment was next, and some tablets to help me through. The rest of the week was a mix of throwing up, not eating, many emotions, dredging up stuff I'd carried around from my childhood and never resolved, not talking, feeling hopeless and lots more intrusive and distressing thoughts. My mind was racing and I couldn't stop it. I felt I'd been doing a pretty good job as a mum up until that point but I now started to question everything. I was particularly anxious that I wouldn't have the good close relationship with my kids that I so desperately wanted.

My thoughts: 'Surely no one could feel this bad? Maybe they'd all be better off if I wasn't here. I'm broken and I can't be fixed. I'm going crazy and they're going to lock me up. I'm never going to feel like myself again'.

Even during these depths, there were many moments of clarity about how ridiculous I was being. Talking about what I was feeling and writing it down really helped but was also deeply confronting and upsetting. And it would take me hours to work up the courage to talk to my husband and/or close friends about what I was really thinking!

The end of the week came and I felt even worse. So, off to the local hospital to be presented with the options: be treated at home or go to one of the few private hospitals that specialise in PND. It was then that I was told just how common PND is.

The trip to the private hospital was long and pretty silent. I wanted to go but was anxious and scared. 'Are there going to be white coats and guards? I wonder if they'll confiscate my shaver? Can I take a hairdryer?'

Being in a psychiatric hospital is the most difficult and confronting thing I've ever done. I find it hard to describe even now. The tears flowed many times during the next four weeks as I started my recovery. It was hard and draining and at times I thought it wasn't doing any good. But I kept telling myself to somehow just hang in there. Good days and not so good days . . . but everyone kept telling me it takes time.

What I experienced at the perinatal hospital (or mums and bubs clinic as I prefer to call it) was an amazing program specifically designed for mums. It focuses on getting mums to a better place, which includes strategies for mums and their babies: group chats, time out for you and lots of other support from experienced and understanding staff, as well as the other great mums in there going down a similar track.

The support for women in my area is excellent. I knew I needed help and put up my hand, but if women don't speak up or the support systems aren't set up or they're migrants or they're poor, then how do they get the right help? Of course there are varying levels of PND and not everyone needs to go to a mums and bubs clinic. The important thing is that PND is demystified so people don't feel ashamed to admit they need help.

Some events in your life stop you in your tracks. The good thing with PND is that it can be treated successfully, although it doesn't happen overnight unfortunately (which is what I wanted!). My journey continues.

Please, have the courage to speak up. You don't have to suffer in silence.

Fay had a different experience, becoming thin-skinned and hyper-irritable. She felt a violence inside her that terrified her. It sat in the pit of her stomach, seeping through her blood and 'filling every limb with rage'. After weeks of little sleep and the near-constant crying of her newborn she was in danger of snapping. Then her toddler, feeling the lack of attention, had a tantrum after Fay had finally succeeded in getting the baby to sleep The baby woke in consequence and Fay lost control:

I bellowed in my toddler's face, grabbed her by the arm and shoved her in her room. Then I rocked the baby back to sleep, hating every minute.

That was the beginning of a downward spiral. I had suffered from the baby blues with my first child but nothing this severe. My husband was working 60-hour weeks, my closest family was an hour away and good reliable friends were busy or elsewhere. Once the rage had escaped there was no turning back. At times I felt the urge to hurt my children. Whenever I had these violent thoughts, I would separate myself from them. I would run to my room and lock them out. Sometimes I would punch my pillows repeatedly, hoping to bash it out. My other outlet was profanity. I barely swore before, but now it was like an addiction. I would curse until I felt I had expelled the anger within. I considered, on numerous occasions, jumping into my car and flattening the accelerator until I was stopped by a tree, a wall or a telegraph pole. I wanted the insanity to end. I believed my family was better off without me. I believed I was losing my mind.

As one who was usually calm I had become the opposite. I felt disconnected from my children, even afraid of them. I resented my husband going to work and leaving me with the kids. I needed help. I wasn't in the right mental state to care for a 17-month-old and a newborn baby. I was so volatile that I kept my distance from them. The television became my toddler's companion. I fed and clothed them but everything else was neglected. Occasionally my sisters would help when they could, but not enough for my needs.

I was in desperate need of respite and aid. I needed to hear a voice of reason. One sister became that voice. I remember feeling separate from myself, as if I was listening to someone else's conversation. I could not believe the words that were forming from my own mouth. I admitted my urge to hurt my children and how sickened I felt by the thought. She answered by stating that I had postnatal depression. She recognised it because she also had endured it with her second child. She encouraged me to see a doctor. I was scared to do that, afraid to admit to it, terrified of owning up to what I had become.

My husband was so stressed with his new position at work and the lack of sleep that he had no energy for us. I needed him, but he wasn't there either. I'd wake to him vomiting in the early morning hours due to stress. Something had to change and quickly. We were both falling to pieces. By grace, my husband received a job offer interstate and he accepted instantly. We stayed with his mother until we found our own home. I hoped she would support me but instead I received criticism. My husband explained that I had postnatal depression but they disregarded it, believing I was incapable and lazy. After six long weeks of living with the in-laws, we acquired our own home. I thought things would improve but I continued to have explosive outbursts and to distrust people.

I forced myself to join a sports group, be social and enjoy my children, yet I felt disconnected from all of them. When I felt like I'd made a breakthrough, I unintentionally sabotaged the success. It was like I was uncontrollably digging a hole and no matter how hard I tried to stop my body kept digging until the hole began to swallow me.

Sometimes my children or my husband would capture my attention. I wanted to go to them, but I just couldn't stop myself from digging the hole deeper. Eventually I knew if I didn't do something I was going to lose my family and myself. I didn't care to a point, but my husband cared and he let me know. It motivated me to fight for them, to get better.

I procrastinated about calling the centres because I felt like such a failure. I felt disappointed that I wasn't the mother I'd envisaged and I was certain others would think the same too—but my family was worth more than my fears. I found some pamphlets and I called the service. I was surprised by the kind reception. I started weekly counselling sessions. My counsellor was very wise and eased my fears. She referred me to a postnatal anxiety group. This group was my saving grace.

The two social workers welcomed me warmly. Child care was provided, as were tea and coffee. For the first time in a long time, I felt nurtured. There were six other women attending the group. We all had reservations about really needing to be there. I was amazed at the mix of women—all intelligent, normal people who were just like me. It comforted me to know I wasn't alone—that I was as normal as they were. We shared our feelings and experiences of our children and our partners, and we were finally understood. We felt fearless in that room. We could honestly say what we needed to say, knowing we wouldn't be judged because of our illogical thoughts. The counsellors offered great advice and broke misconceptions we had on motherhood and ourselves. They offered us confidence and support. When the six-week session was over, I mourned for it. I knew that my support was gone and I would be alone again. However, I took their advice on board.

I started university and took up part-time study. I joined a gym and continued with sports, all of which had child care. My husband helped more around the house and with the children to ease my burden. We made regular date nights to try and bridge the gap that had grown between us. I worked on my assertiveness and low self-esteem. I forced myself to make friends even though I preferred to stay in my hole. I knew that having good people in my life would strengthen me. I arranged to see a psychologist. Group therapy had brought up deeper issues and the counselling helped me think logically about my situation, because logic was an elusive thing during that illness.

Over a period of two years, I managed to overcome my postnatal depression through natural means. I didn't want to be dependent on drugs to balance me out (and I was lucky I didn't have to be). I wanted to develop the life skills necessary to surmount the problem. With consistent effort, I clawed my way out of the hole. It was a struggle, but now I am stronger for it. I understand myself better than before postnatal depression took hold of my life.

THE IMPORTANCE OF TAILORED TREATMENT

Grace, in her essay 'Grace under pressure', asked for a more personalised approach, respecting the fact that the causes and emotions driving the depression are different for every individual:

It's easy to look at the surface symptoms and go 'Hey, that's PND—she's down, she not pasting on a happy smile and pouring cups of tea while breastfeeding at the same time, so it has to be PND . . .' But just as there are different types of cancers, there are different types of depression. It is no good treating the liver if the cancer is in the bowel and it is the same for depression. Every individual must be treated according to the causes and emotions relevant to his or her experience.

This is why I strongly advocate professional psychological help and only using medication to allow yourself a bit of breathing space while you're working through stuff. Luckily, I didn't have a GP who just whacked me on meds and said, 'On your bike, you'll be right.' I am grateful to him for putting me on a mental health plan and referring me to a psychologist, because as much as your family and friends want to help (if you're lucky enough to have this support), they will never be truly impartial or understand.

But getting to a GP was hard in itself. I remember the morning. It was a Sunday. I hadn't had any sleep. I couldn't sleep. It was night after night of being too afraid to go to sleep. I was staying with my mother because it was the only place I felt safe. My poor husband was left in the dark but I didn't know what else to do. Luckily, when I rang the general practice, I was able to see a doctor. I don't remember too much about the visit—I had deteriorated, lost lots of weight and was barely able to hold a conversation.

The doctor prescribed an SSRI antidepressant and sleeping tablets. They were a gift from God! There is a strange perception that if you take antidepressants, you're somehow weak, but people don't seem to share that opinion for coughs and colds, broken legs and back pain. We're supposed to be able to cope with mental and emotional pain and yet, conversely, we know much less about this in Western medicine than we do about physical ailments. I think it's the Australian way: 'She'll be right, mate. Pick y'self up and dust y'self off. No worries.' But there needs to be more talk, more acceptance and more support in this world of illnesses we can't see. Education is vital, to change public perception and unravel myths.

I got better when I began to get sleep, with the help of dedicated grandmothers to assist with feeding through the night. I got better as the meds kicked in. I got better when I worked through my stuff with my psychologist. I got better as I practised the bonding exercises with my daughter.

Now I'm just a regular mum. And my daughter is a regular 2½-year-old. I get fed up some days and want to scream. I still crave 'me' time. But I wouldn't change it for the world. Fortunately, I was able to slowly come off my medication and now I practise yoga regularly, have kinesiology and go to the gym to keep on top of things. I do what I can to maintain a positive state of mind and it's working!

Recognising the specifics of the disorder

We agree that each woman's disorder is composed of different ingredients—a one-size-fits-all model doesn't work. Management for all perinatal disorders *does* have some central components, however—gathering information, seeking help or others seeking help for you, an opportunity to air the distress, practical support at home, de-stressing strategies, normalising sleep, involvement in a support group, and managing risk factors and concerns.

Here is an informal hierarchy of treatment approaches:

- For less severe non-melancholic episodes, non-medication strategies are likely to be the most relevant approach: professional counselling, formal psychotherapy or some other approach that addresses predisposing traits and precipitating stressors.
- For more severe melancholic, psychotic and bipolar disorders, medication is likely to be the initial priority. This may involve some trial and error:
  - Medical practitioners (GPs and psychiatrists) have varying views about which first-line medications to use for these conditions—and an ineffective initial choice may lead to a parade of medications being trialled subsequently.
  - A medication that works rapidly and well for one woman may be ineffective for another, or a medication that has no or few side effects in one woman may produce intolerable side effects in another.

We always reassure people with mood states that are biological (caused by a chemical imbalance rather than stressors) and requiring medication that their condition *can* be brought under control but that we cannot predict whether that will be with the first medication tried, or the second or a subsequent one. In rare cases, hospitalisation may also be appropriate for women with severe episodes of PND. A hospital option may be viewed with dismay by mothers and families, but most facilities do not separate the mother from the baby, treatment and staff skill levels are generally very high, and group camaraderie from a 'band of sisters' also travelling a hard road can be of major benefit.

The vignettes in this chapter capture very severe and high-risk disorders. We chose them so that readers would be aware of the enormous difficulties faced by many women with PND—but often not disclosed to others. Their stories also serve to illustrate the potpourri of biological factors (genetic and medical illness), psychological factors (personality style) and social factors (stressors) that can contribute to perinatal disorders, the differing pathways that helped and—as emphasised throughout this book—that these conditions can be brought under control.

PREVENTING A FUTURE PERINATAL MOOD DISORDER

Child rearing myth: Labour ends when the baby is born.

Anon.

To reduce the risk of any future mood disorder or its recurrence, we recommend putting together a wellbeing plan—drawn up either by you alone or in partnership with your managing health professional. A wellbeing plan allows you to take control of your circumstances rather than feel you're just doing what others have ordered for you.

In formulating a wellbeing plan you should do the following:

- Forgive yourself—you were not or will not be the cause of your perinatal mood condition. Now start afresh.
- Assess any need for medication to maintain a healthy mood.
- Address any marital issues, starting with a discussion about what kind of support you would like from each other.
- Adopt exercise and self-calming or de-stressing strategies such as yoga, mindfulness or meditation.
- Discover therapeutic tools to moderate any aspect of your personality style that makes you vulnerable (such as anxiousness).
- Consider your diet and make gradual healthy changes; take a fish oil supplement.
- Adopt self-nurturing strategies and focus on the simple things in life that provide pleasure.
- Keep a journal to record what worked and what failed to help during the previous episode, the triggers and risk factors, and whether there were any early warning signs. Swift attention may avert another episode.
- Minimise alcohol and stimulants (including avoiding too much caffeine).

- Nominate someone (your partner, or a parent or friend) to provide their observations—only if needed—and who can be called on if there are any signs of an episode brewing.
- List the early warning signs of relapse, discuss them and have a plan of what to do if they emerge.
- Join a support group.
- If you have suffered a puerperal psychosis, there is a risk of recurrence with later pregnancies and so active management and intervention are necessary before and during pregnancy.[2] Select and continue with a competent clinician who can monitor you.

Deciding whether to have another baby

'My son keeps begging for a sister.'

No, your kid is begging for a playmate. Once your child realizes that the loud animal in the Miracle Blanket is his sister he will be appalled and bitter.

Lisa Kilmartin[3]

A key issue for mothers who have experienced an episode of PND is whether to have another child. There is a distinct risk, 20–40 per cent, that those with a past history of perinatal depression will develop an episode during a future pregnancy or after a future birth.[4] This doesn't mean, however, that it is inevitable. You will have noted that many of the essayists in this book reported severe PND with one baby but were untroubled during and after future pregnancies, either naturally or because they took steps to avert another episode. The decision can be made this simply: do you wish to have another baby? Leave any concerns about perinatal depression out of the equation when making that decision.

If you and your partner do decide to have another child, we advise putting some safeguards and supports in place. Set up a support network in advance and lock in help over the first month or so after the birth. Instruct your mother and mother-in-law on what to do, leave a list of important names and phone numbers by the phone, stock the freezer with easily reheated meals, organise children's clothes into categories, and write down the pattern of your family's day so that others can follow your routine. If there's any hint of another episode, ensure that professional help is readily available. And think about having pre-conception counselling from a perinatal psychiatrist (or a general psychiatrist) to discuss your risks of relapse and the best ways to prevent such a relapse, including medication.

eleven

Fathers and the extended family

Appeal from new father: We're not just babysitters, you know. We do try to parent.

Fathers are often overlooked in the saga of pregnancy, childbirth and the first somewhat fraught year. A new dad can be cast mistakenly as a bit character in the unfolding story and feel that he has gone from invincible to invisible. As well as the thrills of new parenthood, there are the spills. For all the joy, it can also be a lonely and isolating time. Most men attest, however, that they are more than ready to step into the role of father.

HOW *DO* FATHERS FIT IN?
Ideally, a father is generally supportive, helping to deal with the increases in washing, housecleaning, shopping and cooking both before and after the advent of the new baby. Ideally, he has the strength to be even more supportive both emotionally and practically if his wife develops a perinatal mood disorder. Some men try to assist but when their usual strategies appear not to work, become overwhelmed and 'disappear', withdrawing mentally and sometimes physically. They are generally still doing paid work, and weariness is not restricted to the new mother. Some new fathers adopt a dispirited trajectory: try to fix the problems at home, work harder, withdraw, drink more or leave altogether. Partners can become the target of the

woman's depression-induced irritability, and may be disinclined to help when all they get is anger in return, thus making the problem even more acute.

Fathers are not immune to PND themselves. Studies estimate that 5–25 per cent are at risk of developing depression during this period. Depressive episodes for partners at this time generally reflect a stress-based response to adapting to parenthood, as well as any losses it represents to their career, relationship and aspirations. Some partners withdraw because they realise they lack the innate resources to be a good and attentive parent and feel (but fail to declare) disappointment in themselves. The risk of depression in a father is increased if his partner has PND.

In turn, women with PND feel a range of emotions about their partner—and his care—at such times. Here are five contrasting experiences:

It is a testament to my husband's strength of character and love that he did what he did during this time. I was little more than a ghost of my previous self. He later told me what a lonely time it was for him. He sees marriage as a team effort, 'Me and you against the world' sort of thing. Initially it had been, but now it was just him and the kids, and this stranger in the house.

Louisa

After about ten months my partner told me he was depressed and had started seeing a counsellor. I felt only anger. I could not complain that he'd stolen this from me; I had not asked for help. But now he was stepping up and claiming the pain for himself. I turned away from him again and refocused on the babies. I hated every day when he came back from seeing the counsellor. I suspected that his sessions were just about criticising me—and part of me could see why he might.

Ivana, the mother of twin girls

Husband is at work. He's always at work. He doesn't have blank walls surrounding him. He has lots of people talking to and around him. He doesn't have silence broken by cries that he is unable to decipher.

He knows exactly what is expected of him, what to expect from others, hears words spoken by colleagues and responds appropriately. There is no time when he stands, with his heart pounding, his ears full of crying and is at a loss. And everything he intends gets done and stays done. He has lunch. He can go to the toilet without background wails to strain his bowels. He doesn't look around his office at piles of mess and clutter and think that it will never move.

Stacey

My husband suffered terribly. He understood nothing but did everything. He grew wings—caring for the children and our home while trying to understand my pain. Thank God he never gave up on me and helped me see it through.

Toula, now a mother of three children

Talia's observations capture how a new baby can provide a moment of truth to a father about his true emotional resources—and diminish his sense of self-worth and drive his own depression:

Whilst our home life was okay, there was certainly underlying stress as can occur when a precious new life arrives front and centre. My husband had a hectic work schedule and started to travel again, coming home frazzled to relay his stressful day to an already exhausted wife. Like many men on overload he often withdraws to cope and finds himself preoccupied with other things, and to a large degree I was emotionally left 'holding the baby'. In hindsight, I understand he really wasn't well enough equipped with emotional resources to allow me to lean on him to the extent I needed and it was a massive learning curve for him, too. During lighter moments we heartily agreed, 'How could something so complex arrive with no manual?'

What's a father to do?

A father carries pictures where his money used to be.

Anon.

Mike and his wife Tessa decided to start a family soon after they married. She quickly became pregnant, 'craving hot chips at all hours of the day and night', and they were thrilled. Mike thought it would be a great time to put the house on the market, as they 'wouldn't be doing much for the next few months'. As he says, 'Big mistake!' At that time he had no idea about the impact a baby might have on their life:

Tessa went into labour on her due date, but it went on and on. The midwife and staff were all reassuring me that everything was okay and how it should be. Me, I'm an engineer—what do I know about having babies? But Tessa was getting distressed. She said to me later that she was unable to communicate her distress and feelings of being out of control. She said, 'I felt absolutely useless. Is a 17-hour labour a "normal" birth?'

At 8.30 that evening, our Tammy-Jean was born. It was a huge celebration for our families: the first grandchild. She was beautiful and in perfect health, big dark-blue eyes, wispy blonde hair. I spent the next few days shuttling between hospital and celebrations with friends and family. It was all a bit of a blur, and such an exciting time of my life. I realised after three days that I hadn't been home. I should feed the dog; he was with our neighbours. Wow, what sort of a parent would I be?

Meanwhile, Tessa was not sleeping well in hospital. She seemed anxious about irrelevant things and still looked pretty washed-out four or five days after the birth. She couldn't eat and was worried about breastfeeding and whether the baby was getting enough milk. I had never seen her like this but assumed it was due to the traumatic birth. The doctor put it all down to exhaustion.

The day we were leaving hospital she suddenly said to me, 'I don't want to come home.' The nurses and I thought it must be the baby blues and she would snap out of it when we got home after some rest, so home we went. I still had another week off work so I thought we'd be able to get into some sort of a routine by then. I realise now that thinking that one week could sort it all out was an indicator of my unrealistic expectations. The baby didn't sleep much, never any longer than an hour or so it seemed; consequently, we tried to take it in turns to get up to her through the night but both of us ended up in zombie mode! Was this normal? We didn't know. And then when Tessa tried to sleep she couldn't relax enough; she was too worried about the baby.

Well, I went back to work and, to be totally honest, I was looking forward to the break away from home—what sort of husband am I? Added to her strain was that people would drop by for a visit. It didn't bother me that the house was messy or chores were piling up. Some of them had new babies themselves and they seemed to be coping fantastically well (which made us feel even more inadequate) but I would notice Tessa put in a massive effort to sound really upbeat and in control while the visitors were there and then be totally exhausted and drained once they left. We talked about these issues but she just couldn't get motivated to do anything, everything was such an ordeal. I think we had too much pride to ask anyone for help and were too embarrassed to admit that we just weren't coping.

Some of my thoughts were: 'Everyone tells us how lucky we are and how happy we should be but we're not!', 'I love Tessa. Why does she hate me!', 'Are we too old for this?', 'I'm the only man on earth in this situation!' The frustration was becoming overwhelming. I could see our life spiralling out of control and I knew this was not normal parenting behaviour. We needed to do something ... but what? I rang the infant healthcare nurse who had been very helpful and asked her if she could visit us, as Tessa wasn't up to visiting the clinic. We felt we could confide in her, and after discussing all of our concerns—not easy—she suggested we get in touch with a GP she knew who specialised in 'PND'—whatever that was! Seriously, I didn't know.

The doctor was wonderful, and for the first time since having the baby we felt like someone understood our situation. She diagnosed Tessa and said she had postnatal depression. I thought, 'What's post-natal depression? So my wife's not crazy. Thank God there's something wrong and some treatment.'

The doctor explained to us that it was a physical imbalance of Tessa's hormones due to the changes in her body from the pregnancy and childbirth and she recommended medication. Her view changed our universe. To not know why you are in such a dreadful, hopeless situation and then to be told that your wife does have a recognised illness that is treatable was the turning point in our little world. Tessa started medication immediately and booked an appointment with a counsellor. I was confident that things would start to improve.

The medication did start to help. After a week or two she was sleeping much better and her whole demeanour seemed to be improving. I felt she was on the road to recovery, but it was very frustrating dealing with an illness that even some medical professionals hadn't heard of or wouldn't acknowledge. We're talking two decades ago, when recognition of the illness called 'PND' was certainly in its own infancy!

Luckily, Tessa's mother was really understanding and helpful. She suggested Tessa and the baby stay with her for a while, she helped out and gave us both a break. It was just what we needed at that stage, and I think it made a big difference to recovery. I couldn't talk to my siblings or friends about it. As much as they cared, they didn't really understand what we were going through. I respected that, as I had no idea what PND was until it had affected us.

Tessa's doctor told us about a group called PANDA that had a presentation night where one of the guest speakers was a fellow talking about his experience of his wife's PND. We attended and it was one of the most interesting speeches I have ever heard. I felt like he was the only other man on earth that would have understood me. It was the boost I needed and made me realise that I could help and support my wife through this until her full recovery. That we would get our great life back we once had.

There is light at the end of the tunnel, and a few months after the diagnosis we were starting to enjoy a lot of things and even having some fun and a few laughs like a normal family. All the little things like writing 'to do' lists and crossing off the most basic tasks to help you get into a positive frame of mind were worth it.

And now, 18 years on, we have a wonderful family (two children), and enjoy life to the utmost. I truly believe that in the long term our

PND experience helped us forge an even stronger relationship that's lasted over 20 years and, believe me, PND has had a positive impact on me personally.

So please don't be afraid or embarrassed to ask for help.

Mike reinforces the messages expressed by mothers in earlier excerpts—the need for sufferers and their families to be aware of and informed about PND, and that a good outcome can be expected, as PND is very responsive to treatment. Mike also underlines two further points: first, the strengths of a marriage are less evident when things are going well and only really emerge when one or both partners are under stress; and secondly, going through the fire can forge an even stronger bond between partners. It certainly leaves enhanced resilience in its wake.

THE STRENGTH OF OTHER FAMILY MEMBERS

Other family members can provide vital assistance to mothers with PND. Your family of origin (your parents and siblings and those of your partner) are so commonly the unsung heroes who provide extraordinary support. Sometimes the extended family is at a loss as to how to provide the best but least intrusive assistance, as the new mother may feel too unsure of herself to engage them. Her partner can perhaps decide with her how to make maximum use of the family's goodwill with minimum exposure to too much well-meaning advice.

Here we note the essential ministrations of Anthea's sister, Tia. She and the rest of the family cradle the new mother until she is able to get back on her feet. In doing this, warmth and affection are also showered on the baby, compensating for Anthea's temporary emotional numbness:

My sister has seen her doctor. My usually bright and voluble sister, I cannot imagine her sitting there with her new daughter in a capsule beside her, telling the doctor how she feels, how she is thinking. Because she is no longer telling any of us.

But it is how I want to imagine it, this unburdening. An unravelling of the tight dark cocoon that has taken her from all of us, leaving her the only one in the family not smiling with unbridled bliss at her daughter.

She manages a phone call most mornings, from her bed. 'Can you come?' She is drowsy with medication and I can hear my niece crying from her bedroom, awake alone in the cot.

'Yes,' I say.

The days are all the same and it is perhaps this that has distressed her, I think, as I lift the baby, change her nappy and dress her. Anthea used to work, living the familiar suburban routine that structures life in so many big cities. Up at six, out the door by seven to catch the train into the CBD, make a date for lunch, explore the city in her breaks, chats with a colleague or a friend. And at five, hanging with the tired slump of every other worker on the train, back to the suburbs, walking her way home, cooking dinner with her new husband, watching television or having friends over to brighten the evenings.

And now evenings are screaming, pacing and aching arms. The tired, strained face of Tony seen over the top of the swaddled baby's head.

I take the baby into the lounge room and lay her on a bright play mat. I adore my niece; she is sunshine and the awakening of life to me. She smiles and I spend hours playing, the games growing outrageous in a bid to keep her laughing, I'm aware that babies need positive interactions. I never tell my sister, but I work hard on my niece's happy patterns. I am only a teenager myself, young and very afraid.

My sister is up and showered, usually, by lunchtime and I make us salad rolls stuffed open with a multitude of vegies. I pour sweet hot tea and take it to her in the lounge room. On a good day I may be able to persuade her on a short walk but not usually, and never to the park where other happy mothers may make demands on what she 'ought' to be feeling by their very presence, their boastful attentiveness to their babies, their washed hair, ironed clothes and cheery exchanges. Even their plastic toys are an affront in the dark tunnel where Anthea is stuck.

My sister is a sad blob. We dance around her, my niece and I, but our smiles and chuckles elicit no response. She is staring at the television: endless soap operas and talkback programs.

We are no strangers to depression, my sister and I. It is part of our history, part of the family story—dad, grandad, uncles. But never the women. My mother urges busyness, doing things even if you don't feel like it, getting out, socialising. Distraction. She has weathered many episodes with my father.

But this is different. There is a baby, a new marriage, a young husband. The expectations on my sister are enormous. Sitting in her house, alone with her in the suburbs—mortgage, marriage, pets, parenting—I can feel obligations pressing in on both of us. Even the nappy packet's jolly picture is offensive.

Despair?

We never leave her alone, not for a whole day.

I look at the empty saucepans and fill them with prepared vegetables, ready on the stove. Tony can take it from there when he gets home.

* * *

None of us is prepared for the return of animation when it comes. It starts slowly, but is unmistakable, like watching rocks crack over bright lava, knowing the release of steam is a sign of change. Change. A PANDA meeting: Anthea's relief is palpable. She has sat in as part of a circle of women who are all feeling as she feels, expressing things she is expressing. She is excited, talking, animated. Gradually, the effect wears off. Once she has told each of us about the meeting, she slides into her usual position either on the bed or armchair. But then there is another meeting, and this time she visits the PANDA offices between meetings, she makes a private appointment, the house fills with shiny white brochures with a logo of the calmly munching PANDA bear. Lists begin to appear under magnets on the fridge. As time goes on she says the medication is really helping her and the side effect of morning drowsiness causes irritation, not indifference. I secretly rejoice. Then she is arguing—arguing!—giving her viewpoint about her experience, her need for support from her husband

and demanding he attend groups designed for men so as to educate himself about PND.

She is taken on many breaks, always with others to care for the baby, now almost a year old. I have two photographs from these trips. In the first, Anthea is overweight, morose, looking away into the distance from a bench by the sea, her baby beside her in a pram, ignored. In the second, her hair is windswept and she is leaning into her husband on a pier, laughing and teasing.

Anthea's second experience of motherhood is all the better for her being a woman returned from a long dark and lonely journey, a mother finding deep gratitude in having survived the black dog the first time around and feeling doubly joyful in the realisation that he isn't returning this time as she dreaded. I watch her pleasure mingled with disbelief as she becomes the mother she always wished and imagined herself to be.

And I feel that all of us have faced it down together, that baby black dog.

Here is a final observation—expressed from a child's viewpoint (though written decades later). It reflects earlier years when the big 'D', depression, was not mentioned—to children or to others. Just getting on with things was a strategy when little to no effective treatment was available. Natural remission, if the woman was lucky, was the order of the day.

The writer fashions fragments of memories into a picture in 'When your mother was unwell':

My sister was born on a Wednesday morning in a hospital room with lemon curtains. In the moments before, the doctor on duty rolled up his sleeves and washed his hands, then polished his silver instruments. At half past ten, he said, 'It's time.' But my sister, as if aware of what would follow, decided to stay back.

For 45 minutes, in fact.

When she finally emerged, fist clenched and face as creased as a tea towel, the doctor hung her upside down and slapped her for keeping him waiting. Then a nurse with silver hair carried her over to the sink and another, a little younger, washed her in a bowl of olive oil. After they cut her cord, they put her on a cooking scale. My sister was smaller than the rest of us, only 5 pounds [2.25 kilograms]—the weight of a bluebird, or a bag of apricots.

When he was contacted, my father shuffled us into the car and brushed down our hair and buckled our seatbelts. Then he went searching for an empty car space—one with shade so the wheel would not warm—and after that for a ticket machine and loose change and a payphone so he could call the bowls club.

'I need to cancel my roll-up,' he said.

By the time we arrived on the second floor, my mother was sitting on the edge of her bed, white-faced and hair wet, gown off one shoulder. My father hurried to her side.

'She's got my nose,' he said, touching his own.

My mother nodded.

'She's smaller than I expected,' he said, 'but we'll keep her.'

My mother looked out the window. 'Something's wrong,' she said.

My father drove us home.

A couple of days later, the jacaranda in our backyard started to bloom; its purple trumpets fell from the sky and dotted our lawn, and my mother came home from hospital. She put the baby on the bench and told my father she was going to lie down. Before bed, she stood at the sink and sipped a glass of water. Then she held my face between her hands and said, 'Mummy isn't well.' For the rest of my life I would feel, unexplainably, that I needed to make her better.

That night my father tucked us in.

The next morning, and for many mornings after that, I woke to the sound of someone crying. At first I thought the crying belonged to the baby because it started at sunrise before the birds and it seemed like all cries came from a child. Except after a while I realised the crying was not from the baby.

One morning I opened the door to my parents' room and saw them lying in bed together, my father flat on his back, my mother curled over him like a starfish. Her head was on his chest and her eyes were red and puffy. My father reached for a handkerchief from the lowboy and unfolded it. For a second our eyes met and he looked at me as if to say, 'Close the door.'

In the months that followed my brother and I would spend entire hours, sometimes days, with our ears against the walls. In the crying world, far from the playful sounds of school, we wondered what would happen to us. My father I think sensed these ruffles in our thoughts and tried to smooth them over.

'Everything is fine,' he said.

At night he let us cook popcorn with extra salt and butter and in the morning we went on adventures. On school days we drove through McDonald's and ordered bacon and eggs. My father, unsure what to feed the growing baby, took a hash brown from its packet and blew on it till it was cold. I squashed out the lumps and passed bits to my brother. He fed her, piece by piece.

'She loves it,' he reported. 'Give me more.'

Eventually, we called my sister 'Tot'.

After school we went to the bowls club. My father watched us over a beer. When he wasn't looking we fed our sister potato chips from a plastic cup. Other times we let strangers tickle her feet.

'Where's your mother?' one of them asked.

'We don't have a mother,' my brother said.

'Nonsense.'

'Our mother's in the circus,' I said.

That afternoon, someone reported our family to the manager and we weren't allowed back. On the way out, my father took me aside. 'The circus?' he said. 'Is that the best you could do?' As we spoke, my brother climbed a tree and started shaking the branches. 'I'm a monkey,' he said. My father shook his head and said, 'You're an idiot.' Then he started joining in.

When we were older my father would refer to this time simply as 'when your mother was unwell'. When we started high school we complained about cereal for breakfast. 'We used to get McDonald's,' we said. 'That was a long time ago,' my father said, 'when your mother was unwell.'

It was around this time, after the monkey incident, that my aunts came to live with us. There were five of them all up, one for each day of the week.

'Monday's here,' my brother would call, 'and she's got Thursday with her.'

Our aunts emptied the cupboards and watered the plants and scrubbed the floors with hot water and disinfectant. They came with suggestions and bottles of tablets, and they tried to make sense of my mother's closed door. They made her so many cups of tea that long after they left I found mugs scattered in obscure places.

In the weeks that followed, the colour returned to my mother's cheeks from wherever it had disappeared to. Slowly she started to feel better. To speed her recovery the doctor suggested she spend some time in a clinic apart from us. My mother complained to my father about the space between us but he was a man of reason who grew up to the ticking of a clock and he believed if something was ordered then it was acceptable.

'This will work,' he said.

The next day, my mother packed up all her things and told us she was going away for a while. Before she left she sat us at the kitchen table and poured our cordials and cut our sandwiches into perfect squares.

'When I'm gone be good for your father,' she said.

'Where are you going?'

My mother picked up her keys. 'I'm going on a little holiday,' she said.

'Can we come?'

'I would take you if I could,' my mother said, 'but children aren't allowed.'

Later that night my mother came home in a police car. From my window I saw the officer help her out of the car. For a while she stood under the streetlight straightening out her dress. My father, who was waiting in the lounge room, met them at the door. They spoke in low voices but through their muffled conversation I could still make out some words.

'Maybe three or four hours,' one of them said.

'Yes, the Gateway Bridge.'

After that, my father kept the car keys in his drawer.

Days passed and seasons changed and for a long time things stayed the same. My father went to work and my mother went back to bed. Neighbours called with news and meals, my aunts came and went.

Spring returned, the jacaranda bloomed again, my sister learned to walk.

Then one Tuesday, on a morning as ordinary as any other, my mother got out of bed. She straightened the sheets and plumped up the pillows and ran her hand along the edge of the bed. She gave my father a little shake but he grumbled and rolled the other way.

She stood in the bathroom and called our names as if they were words she had forgotten. She put us in the bathtub one by one and scrubbed our hands and feet. She soaped our hair and dried us off and said sweet soothing things like, 'It's all right.'

Eventually my father woke and got up and found us in the backyard. The four of us were sitting legs crossed in the shade of the jacaranda. My brother was digging holes and my mother was filling them. My sister was eating some dirt.

'Is everything okay?' my father asked.

'We're planting a new tree,' my brother said.

My father looked over at my mother.

'I feel better,' she said.

RAISING THE SUBJECT OF SEEKING HELP

You're a partner, a family member or a good friend. You can see that the new mother is not herself and hasn't been for some time. How do you tactfully suggest that she seek assistance from a health professional? And how do you bring this up without making things worse?

There is no one strategy but here are some options to consider. Many of these recommendations are drawn from the book *Living with a Black Dog* by Matthew and Ainsley Johnstone.[1]

Seeking advice

It is useful to consult someone with experience and knowledge of perinatal mood disorders. Why? First, it helps to have a better grasp of what you think is happening. Secondly, it can make your own thoughts clearer before you broach the subject. Thirdly, it helps you decide what you want to get out of the discussion. How you come across to the mother-to-be or the new mum is very important; ideally she'll see you as a strong, reassuring presence and gain a clear view of what you would like to see happen and the acceptable alternatives.

Many people are concerned that to intervene is to be intrusive. If a friend was showing signs of a physical problem you would probably express concern, so raising your concern about an intimate's mental health issue should not be viewed as crossing a line—rather, it demonstrates that you care.

Broaching the subject

You probably know the situations when you feel most comfortable together. Or you can create a time when you can talk together without pressure or interruption. Decide how far you want to press the subject—there's likely to be resistance or denial at first. If it's too difficult, now that you've opened up the subject, you could suggest a future time for raising your concerns again.

What to say and how

You can let her know what you've noticed and why you're concerned. You are a familiar contact to her, but that may not make it any easier to raise a sensitive subject that's so close to her sense of self and her competence. Paradoxically, the fact that she has lost her bearings and you have noticed may initially make her alarmed and defensive.

What she will want is your support. Try to take things at her pace and respect her point of view. Validate what she says and try not to reassure by minimising her distress. Listen attentively and resist giving advice, let alone judgement. If she has lost touch with reality, you can convey that you understand that what she is experiencing is real for her but that you see things a different way—and that consulting a professional is a step towards reducing her stress and sorting things out so that she can enjoy motherhood.

Deciding if an assessment is needed

Hopefully, your gut feelings will tell you whether the woman you're concerned about simply needs support or a break and a lightening of her load to allow her time out to recharge. If you make that judgement, review what's happening within a week to check that she was not simply putting on a brave face and covering up a more substantial and persisting perinatal mood condition.

If assessment is warranted, consider the best first option. Any assessment should be discreet and sensitive and agreed to by the mother. Don't ambush her. A mothercraft nurse who has been recommended by others can visit and give some pointers about feeding and settling the baby. This would be an acceptable intervention, and the nurse could then make an independent judgement about the need for additional assessment. If consulting a GP, ensure you find one who's sympathetic—perhaps, but not necessarily, a female practitioner who has had children. Ask the receptionist to book a longer appointment and, if possible and acceptable, accompany the mother to the appointment. The doctor may see the woman by herself first and then invite you in later or, if the mother prefers, you might sit in on the whole interview. You need to be the ears: if the mother is distressed she may not hear much of what the clinician has to say.

At the end of an assessment you will have a sense of the professional's judgement and your instinct can be useful. Your priority is to leave with a detailed and comprehensive assessment, a diagnosis (such as depression or another, even physical, condition, or further tests to clarify), the causes of her condition and the recommended management options.

There may not be a clinical problem at all. Even if this is the case, the discomfort and worry you felt is most likely resolved through talking with someone like a counsellor skilled in the area who has seen it all before.

Why not just wait it out?

Waiting out a woman's distress during the perinatal time is *never* the best option. Untreated depression or anxiety is distressing to the woman, disruptive to the family's wellbeing and, while it persists, can compromise the mother–child bond.

twelve

Mothers' strategies

Here is a collection of the best tips provided by mothers.

A GOOD GP

While pregnant, find yourself a nearby GP who you click with. This is your new best friend. You can download on them during the odd day when it's all a bit much! A good GP is tolerant and reassuring of your worries and actually welcomes your visits when you have concerns about the new baby or your other little ones. Check that your doc is likely to be staying on at that practice and that they work near to full-time (so that they are there when you need them).

CRYING, CRYING, CRYING

Babies sometimes cry for no discernible reason yet we're hard-wired to try to fix it for them. Have a checklist to reassure yourself that you've done what you can, ensure that there's no high temperature or obvious illness, then have a list of circuit breakers to help you: take him/her for a walk where the crying doesn't matter, maybe earphones and music for a while, use the car and put on your CD, give the baby a bath or a massage, ring a helpline so they can soothe you, exercise vigorously for ten minutes in the next room.

RAINING, RAINING, RAINING

Cabin fever, cramped quarters, and everything damp! Take off to the shopping mall or the library; get a friend with a littlie to come to you; if you have a car it can be a mobile room—a favourite CD of songs and rhymes and a few snacks and treats—a change of scene. Treat yourself to the local laundry's dry-and-fold service.

TIPZZZ ABOUT SLEEP

My babies liked to be tightly wrapped: they're regular little Houdinis! The commercial wraps designed to keep the baby from unwrapping itself are a worthwhile investment. Stuff a comforter down your front during the day to give it your smell and then tuck it over the fitted sheet for the baby to sleep on. A rhythmic 'ssshing' noise can help to settle them—I used to do it while rocking or patting the baby but avoiding eye contact so that he got the message that it was sleep time. Keep stimulation down during night feeds: just enough dim lighting to feed the right end of the baby and to avoid broken toes from the ever-present bouncinette. This helps the baby to distinguish night from day and learn that night feeds are just that and then it's straight back to bed.

Please accept help (like I didn't). Your partner/family can watch the baby so you can sleep/shower/eat. Grab sleep whenever you can—even 15 minutes helps. Find out your baby's tired signs (for example, jumping jack agitated arm and leg movements and avoiding eye contact with you) and put them down for a nap as soon as those signs appear. Overtired babies are harder to settle.

Some babies only need 45-minute naps in the day once they are no longer newborns (old wives' tales say the less they sleep the brighter they are—but certainly that doesn't apply to the mum!).

If the baby's having a bad night, share the load with your partner. Take turns at getting three to four hours' sleep while the other settles the bub. If it's too exhausting for you and you're breastfeeding, your partner may be able to give the occasional bottle-feed at night—my baby girl wouldn't take a bottle from me, only from my husband, as she knew I had 'the goods'. (BTW, both my babies would fuss at the breast if I'd been out and smelled different because I'd put on perfume for an occasion!)

DIFFICULTIES WITH BIRTH, AND ITS AFTERMATH

Birth versus baby: There is so much focus on the birth plan (which nearly always bears no relation to what happens) that everyone forgets the birth is simply the preliminary for a baby. Prepare for this eventuality: for instance cook and freeze meals, gather handy tips from the nurses, look at what groups and supports are available in your area, etc. Don't just buy more stuff for the nursery.

My career as a registered nurse (in operating theatres where I witnessed many caesarean sections) taught me that delivery of a healthy baby by the safest means is the ultimate goal. A colleague once said, 'You don't have a baby to have a birth . . . you have a baby to have a family.' This was an invaluable comment for me. While a natural delivery is to be hoped for, I felt no pressure to idealise the type of birth I had.

Birth is rightly called 'labour'. Many women are a bit shell-shocked after and some relive the experience, even to the extent of experiencing PTSD. See your GP for advice. He or she can ensure that there are no lingering physical problems and perhaps recommend a counsellor to deal with any recurring feelings and settle you.

An appeal: Can paediatricians, in particular, be given more training in identifying and managing PND? My baby was born with disabilities but despite all the specialists checking him, not one ever looked up from the cascade of abnormal test results to see that I was hanging by a thread. A motherly nurse at one of the clinics took the time to find me some support.

You need some talks while you're still in hospital to make you aware of the types of resources available and for what situations, or at least a handout to take away to read. The hospitals should be the first people to educate mums that it's okay to ask for help.

WHAT ABOUT SEX?

There's a bit of a conspiracy of silence about differences in libido at this time. It's surprising that with all the talk about the physicality of birth and breastfeeding, one of the most disrupted bonds at this time is that of sex between the mother and father of the baby. Dr Martien Snellen's book Rekindling: Your Relationship after Childbirth *(Text Publishing, 2010) is helpful. Maybe the parents of the new babe can seek a joint counselling session where they can both raise concerns if problems persist.*

DIFFICULTIES WITH BREASTFEEDING

Your baby health centre, friends and mothercraft nurses at the hospital are all likely to have good advice or contacts to help you establish breastfeeding. Persist if you can; most women take a while to get the hang of it. [There is also a list in Chapter 8 of the websites of organisations (including the Australian Breastfeeding Association) that have helplines.] *The axiom is 'breast is best' but if you wish or need to bottle-feed, do not feel lingering guilt or a sense of failure. You have your own good reasons for your decision. Your baby will thrive.*

SOMETHING FOR EVERYONE

- *We told everyone we were having a 'babymoon' when we came back from hospital. Say that you'll be keeping very much to yourselves for the first ten days (phone off the hook), and not to feel excluded as you'll have one big get-together three weeks after the homecoming when everyone can visit all at once.*
- *Remember that being intellectually prepared (with oodles of pre-reading) is not the same as being emotionally prepared. That can't really happen until you walk in your front door and find yourself totally in charge of a newborn. It's a steep learning curve for a while but hang in there; each day makes a difference. Ask for help if you need it.*

- *Shape it up for those who offer help so that they know how to provide it most efficiently: a balance between what you want and what they can do.*
- *Just before bed do as much as you can to get ready for the next day. Set the table for breakfast, lay out clothes for yourself and the baby, maybe put on a load of washing to be ready for the line next day.*
- *Try to restrict housework to the essentials, for instance sort the baby's stuff out enough and ahead of time to prevent the next task from becoming a frustrating muddle.*
- *Accept cooked meals that you can freeze and defrost when needed. Suggest at your baby shower that the gift you want is for everyone to pledge one meal for your first weeks at home with the new baby.*
- *Write a list of what you like to do and where you can do it. When you're sleep deprived you'll find that both inspiration and motivation can sag. You can refer to your list at the beginning of such mornings. It might include time-fillers that are cheap and accessible at the local shopping centre, the more toddler-friendly cafes to visit or where you can see friends, some rainy weather activities/ places that worked for you or others.*
- *Writing, be it a journal or a record of the cute things the baby does, helps make sense of everything!*
- *Record the usual routine you follow with the baby: nappy change routine, usual wake/sleep times, bottles and formula instructions if relevant. That way someone else can shoulder some of the load occasionally. Keep a list of all the important phone numbers beside the phone, too.*
- *Break your day into four segments to differentiate it, with maybe one thing you should do and one thing you want to do in each. Mark the chunks of time with a cuppa, a sit-down, some time to yourself when possible so it doesn't seem endless.*
- *Look up internet sites that describe the developmental milestones for each month of a baby's life. This information transforms what can look like a feeding and excreting machine into a little human being that, in front of your eyes, becomes a little more independent*

each week. Online resources and support, mums' groups and mummy blogs can go some way to lessen isolation, especially if you're new to town. The local library has computers if you don't have access to one at home.

- *In the last weeks of pregnancy buy in a packet of thank-you cards and a jotter. After coming home with your baby, keep a scribbled list of who should be thanked for what and then get a girlfriend to copy in a fairly standardised note that you can sign. She can address and post the envelopes.*

- *Don't waste time doing housework. Let it go! Or if that worries you too much, keep one 'reception' room tidy. Have a couple of packets of fancy biscuits in reserve: this is no time for making cakes.*

- *Ditch the cape, Superwoman! You can re-don it when they start school . . . or maybe never.*

- *Playing with your baby is NEVER wasting time. Your touch and gaze, your smile and your response to their needs (even when you can't figure out what they want!) is pure gold. Follow their lead when you can.*

- *Try to 'stay with' your child while they are managing an intense feeling (for example, frustration). Later you might want to talk about that situation to help them recognise and share their feelings.*

- *If you have more than one baby and they are look-alikes, a dab of nail polish on a toe can help you pick one from the other.*

- *If you go to a supportive mothers' group (not a competitive one) ask whether you can have a regular ten-minute brainstorming session that contributes mums' best ideas for settling, feeding and other day-to-day realities.*

- *My toddler (now 15!) used to throw terrific tantrums. I'd be so embarrassed, imagining what people were saying (probably didn't even notice—just moved away from the wails . . .). What I found best was the parents' room/baby-change bathroom. Most shopping malls have one. We'd dash in there and I'd shelter until his storm had passed.*

- *It's obvious but being a new mum is hard work and in reality no one looks like those women in the television commercials. As well, all the other mums look as if they're managing better than you. That's a fairy tale too.*

- *I get easily irritated so I have to use some tricks to top up my 'patience quotient'. I say to myself, 'Sam [my baby] hasn't woken up on purpose just to stop me doing [fill in blank]' and 'I'm the adult here and I can understand that my baby is just . . . being a baby.' I also repeat to myself: 'I'm bigger, stronger, wiser and kind.' When I'm getting really frayed I literally put my fingers in my ears, take deep breaths and slowly count to ten.*

- *There are going to be days when you 'know' you're a hopeless mother. You're not. You're the only mother your baby knows and wants.*

- *There's too much unhelpful advice given too forcefully. Smile and look vague and grateful . . . and follow your own instincts.*

- *Pamper yourself with a facial or massage. Get your husband to look after the baby for half an hour while you have a bubble bath. Keep a diary of the funnier or sadder things that happen over the weeks.*

- *Try not to get too caught up in the fervent quasi-religious beliefs that surround birth and breastfeeding. Be as pragmatic as you can be about what works for you and your baby.*

- *Get fresh air during the day. Take the baby for a walk whenever you can. My partner bundles me out the door nearly every morning so that I can have a walk or jog or even just a coffee for 45 minutes by myself before he leaves for work*

- *Plans that involve other people or specific times need to be flexible: keep people's phone numbers handy so you can change arrangements at a moment's notice*

- *If you're not managing, practise self-acceptance and have the courage to reach out for help. Be kind to yourself. Don't overload yourself. How can you give and give to your baby if you don't first give to yourself and allow yourself time to recharge?*

- *If you score the unlucky door prize, postnatal depression, reframe it (when you get your head back), not as a weakness but as an opportunity to gain strength.*

- *If you need treatment for postnatal depression take responsibility for it. You are in the driver's seat.*

- *Please, you can recover; and you're not alone!*
- *If you need medication, be pragmatic. Your GP can outline an approach and refer you to a specialist for more detailed advice and management. Medication is not addictive and if it's needed to treat your mood disorder, you'll be the better mother because of it. Be patient if there's some trial and error before the best medication or combination is achieved.*
- *I got great help from our neighbour's school-age daughter who was my extra pair of hands between 4 and 6 pm, dealing with the toddler while I bathed and fed the baby. Surprisingly, it made me much more patient with everything. She loved the extra pocket money, too.*
- *Returning to work part-time may be of benefit in regaining an identity outside of being a mother. The cost of child care may consume most of your earnings but remember, that's not the point.*
- *If you're a bit short of money, op shops have fabulous things, especially kids' clothes and lucky finds in toys. The community centre in your suburb lists activities that are free or affordable; a park with a jungle gym plus a picnic, a bubble wand and some bread for the birds can do the trick; the local shopping mall has space where you can meet friends and sit with a takeaway coffee (a treat tucked away and offered at the right time can distract the littlie's attention from toyshops or food outlets or a threatened tantie). The library has free activities and will look up free or cheap outings for you. Ring your local council about activities and playgroups.*

Appendix

Medications in the perinatal period

Some women planning to have a baby are already on psychotropic medication—antidepressant medication for depression, anxiety or even to assist sleep, or a mood stabiliser or an antipsychotic drug (to treat a bipolar disorder or to augment an antidepressant medication). Women commonly ask, 'Is this medication safe to take while I'm pregnant or while I breastfeed?' Here are some answers.

UNDERSTANDING RISK VERSUS BENEFIT

There's no straightforward answer to the question of whether medication is safe during pregnancy and breastfeeding. In all cases, the risk of potential harm to the developing foetus must be balanced against the benefits to a mother who is more functional when taking medication. Any analysis of risk versus benefit must therefore consider the downsides of ceasing medication (such as increased potential for relapse of the illness). If you have suffered from a perinatal mood disorder before, this discussion should ideally take place with your doctor before you become pregnant but, if not, as soon as possible after your pregnancy has been confirmed.

Risks versus benefits of medication during pregnancy				
	Not taking medication		Taking medication	
	Benefits	Risks	Benefits	Risks
Mother	—	Risk of relapse of depression or bipolar disorder	Maternal wellbeing	Side effects of medication
Developing foetus	No risk of harm from medication	Risk of impact of severe depression on foetal development	Reduced risk of impact of severe depression on foetal development	Risk of harm from exposing foetus to medication

Possible effect of medication during each trimester of pregnancy

- *First trimester exposure*—potential for particular foetal malformations, pregnancy loss or miscarriage.
- *Second trimester exposure*—impact on foetal growth rate, size for gestational age, birth weight.
- *Third trimester exposure*—effects on birth weight, size for gestational age; risks of pulmonary hypertension in the newborn (PPHN; see below) or of neonatal abstinence syndrome (NAS; see below).

Information about medication effects: registers and TGA categories

Research into the safety of medications in pregnancy together with side-effect data is collected in registers and collated into categories. Registers such as MotherSafe (Australia) or MotherRisk (Canada) determine whether specific drugs taken during pregnancy increase the risk of congenital abnormalities. They also collect information on the subsequent development of children exposed to such drugs during pregnancy or breastfeeding.

Contact these registers (their websites are listed at the end of this appendix) for detailed information and advice.

In Australia, all medicines are categorised by the Therapeutic Goods Administration (TGA) for their safety in pregnancy. There are five categories (A–D and X), as outlined in the box below.

TGA CATEGORIES FOR SAFETY OF MEDICATIONS IN PREGNANCY

Ways to find out out how the medication is classified:

1. Ask a GP or pharmacist; they will have access to the MIMS guide that gives the classification.
2. Safety in pregnancy and breastfeeding findings are provided on the Product Information sheet that can be downloaded from the TGA website. This information is NOT provided in the Consumer Medicine Information (that is, it's not on the package insert included with the medication).

- *Category A* medications have been taken by large numbers of pregnant women and who have shown no ill effects. In consequence, such medications are considered safe to use during pregnancy and breastfeeding.
- *Category B* medications have been taken by fewer pregnant women. They have not shown any increased frequency of malformation or other direct or indirect harmful effects on the foetus. Such medications are subclassified according to whether or not animal studies can provide additional safety information.
- *Category C* medications have caused, or are suspected of causing, harmful (reversible or irreversible) effects on the human foetus without causing malformations.
- *Category D* medications are suspected of causing harm to the developing foetus.
- *Category X* medications should not be taken by pregnant women or in circumstances where there is a possibility of pregnancy.

Medication categories and safety

As many medications have only come onto the market in the last decade and as large registers are required to exclude—rather than simply confirm—any medication risk, most medications used in psychiatry are either category B or C (in other words, no firm statement can be made about their safety during pregnancy), except for the mood stabilisers, which are listed as category D drugs.

For those psychotropic medications where there does appear to be sufficient data, there appear to be only very small risks to the developing foetus. Several others carry a greater risk, as reflected in their TGA classification.

There is always a risk that *any* newborn infant will have a congenital abnormality. Around 2 per cent—that is, two babies in every 100 born—will have something wrong with them. This is illustrated in the figure below. The sad faces represent infants with an abnormality.

Risk of a foetal abnormality per 100 pregnancies

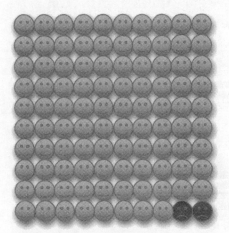 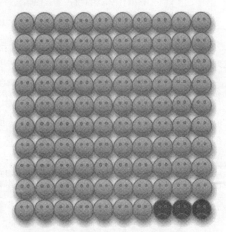

There is about a 2 per cent risk for healthy women of having a baby with a congenital abnormality

There is about a 3 per cent risk for women who have been taking an antidepressant of having a baby with a congenital abnormality

If the mother is taking an SSRI (selective serotonin reuptake inhibitor) antidepressant, there is a slightly increased risk of harm to the foetus: three out of 100 foetuses exposed to an SSRI may have an abnormality, such as a mild heart defect. Despite this slightly increased risk above the baseline (that is, from 2 to 3 per cent), the risk posed by taking this medication may be acceptable if there is clear benefit to the mother.

A CHECKLIST FOR BEFORE AND DURING PREGNANCY AND AFTER THE BIRTH

Discuss any intention to reduce or cease your medication with your doctor. To avoid serious withdrawal effects from abrupt cessation, and to avoid the possibility of relapse of illness, it is essential to work out a safe regime for withdrawing from your medication gradually.

Find a good (and readily available) GP, preferably one with an interest in mental health as well as in mothers and babies. If there are significant risks from any medication you are taking you will need your doctor's advice and monitoring.

Your doctor should also:

- take a thorough history of your background, your present situation and aspects of your mental and physical health
- possibly collaborate with your obstetrician and paediatrician
- discuss with you the risks versus the benefits of continuing or tapering your current medications (including herbal or alternative medications such as St John's wort) and even initiating different psychotropic medications
- assess your support network
- advise you on health-related activities and offer any local supports for you for during your pregnancy and after the birth if judged to be useful.

PSYCHOTROPIC MEDICATION DURING PREGNANCY AND BREASTFEEDING

Most medications used to treat depression or bipolar disorder pass across the placenta and through to the developing foetus. Some also pass though breastmilk. Ever since the tragedy of thalidomide there have been concerns about the effect of medications on the developing foetus—that they could interfere with the development of body organs, particularly the heart, and especially over the first trimester. There is a risk of adverse impacts later in pregnancy as well.

Mothers and psychotropic medication

Tell your treating doctors (including your obstetrician), as well as the midwife, about any medication you're taking. They should tell you whether it is possible you will experience any side effects and, if so, their likely impact on your wellbeing during your pregnancy. They should also tell you whether the medication could have an adverse effect on the course of your pregnancy.

Extensive research into the effects of medication on the foetus during pregnancy, and later on the newborn and the growing child, is complicated by the fact that some poor outcomes are more the result of other factors during pregnancy, such as smoking, poor diet and poor antenatal care.

Overall, studies of psychotropic medication effects on mothers have not found major problems with pregnancy outcomes, but research has highlighted some concerns, two of which are: a possible increased risk of high blood pressure associated with the SSRI antidepressants, and excessive weight gain and gestational diabetes associated with the newer antipsychotic medications (which are sometimes used as mood stabilisers for women with bipolar disorder).

Antipsychotic medications in pregnancy

- Older (typical) antipsychotic medications are generally considered by experienced clinicians to be safe during pregnancy and are often used to treat nausea and vomiting in pregnancy.
- Newer, second-generation (atypical) antipsychotic medications can contribute to weight gain and increase the risk of a mother developing gestational diabetes.

The registers (see above) offer insufficient data to make a firm statement about the safety of both of these groups of medications, and most typical and atypical antipsychotic medications have been classified by the TGA as Category C.

Mood stabilisers in pregnancy

The mood stabilisers present a particular difficulty, as their risks during pregnancy are variable. They are important, however, in treating women with bipolar disorder, who have a high risk (at least 50 per cent) of relapse following childbirth if they remain untreated. Here are some specifics:

- Lithium was considered to increase the risk of a specific heart defect and so was long viewed as contraindicated in pregnancy. While that risk is now known to be low, the use of lithium is not recommended. As ceasing lithium (or any other mood stabiliser) can lead to a bipolar relapse, such medication should be tapered off slowly over a few months.
- Lithium passes through the placenta. Although it can be used again later in the pregnancy, it must be carefully monitored to ensure the correct dose, and the dose must then be lowered later in the pregnancy to prevent the baby experiencing side effects.
- Sodium valproate (Epilim) is used as a mood stabiliser but is not recommended for women of childbearing age. It has been linked with a high risk of congenital abnormality (about 17 per cent), and adverse effects on foetal brain development that put the baby at risk of developmental delay.
- Lamotrigine is considered to be one of the safer mood stabilisers during pregnancy, but as the registers have only small databases on this medication, it is listed as a Category D drug.

Psychotropic medication and breastfeeding

- Most of the medications used to treat depression are safe for the breastfeeding infant but their dose and some potential complications should be discussed with the managing doctor or a lactation consultant. Such a discussion should of course weigh risks against benefits.
- These medications do pass through breastmilk to the feeding infant so the prescribing doctor should calculate the relative infant dose (RID). A rule of thumb is that the level of medication in breastmilk should be less than 10 per cent of its level in the mother's blood for it to be considered safe for breastfeeding to continue. The doctor should take this into account when determining the dose.
- The safety of psychotropic medication depends on how well the infant is able to metabolise it (that is, get rid of it), as a young baby's liver is not fully mature and cannot deal with

some medications or is less efficient at doing so, which means they can then build up and cause side effects.

- Some medications are not recommended for breastfeeding mothers—lithium passes though the breastmilk and into the baby. In light of potential harmful side effects to the baby it is contraindicated for breastfeeding mothers. The safety during breastfeeding of lamotrigine (used to treat bipolar disorder) is unknown.
- As a woman with a bipolar disorder risks relapse if her medication is ceased, this outweighs the benefits of breastfeeding, so she would be advised to bottle-feed her infant.

Antidepressants during pregnancy and breastfeeding

- A review of the scientific literature[1] indicated that antidepressants may slightly increase the risk of miscarriage and of a lower birth weight (the latter through a slightly increased risk of pre-term delivery).
- The commonly used SSRI antidepressants slightly increase the risk of heart defects in the infant. One study[2] analysed data from five meta-analyses (which aggregate findings from smaller studies): four did not find increased risk of foetal malformations in the first trimester of pregnancy for mothers taking SSRIs, while one found a slight increased risk of cardiac malformations in infants exposed to the SSRI paroxetine.
- The same study found that, though fewer reports had examined the SNRIs (serotonin norepinephrine reuptake inhibitors— such as venlafaxine, desvenlafaxine and mirtazapine), there did not appear to be evidence that they increased the risk of congenital defects.
- There are only minimal data for some other antidepressant medication classes, but absence of evidence does not mean evidence of absence (that is, that there are no associated risks) for the newer antidepressants.
- The SSRIs and other antidepressants slightly increase the risk of elevated blood pressure in the mother during pregnancy.[3]
- The SSRIs may increase the risk of persistent pulmonary

hypertension in the newborn (PPHN), a rare condition (occurring in about one baby per 20,000) that is somewhat more likely to occur or persist for a period when the mother has taken an SSRI during late pregnancy (though it may be associated with earlier use during pregnancy).

- The newborn may go through a withdrawal syndrome called Poor Neonatal Adaptational Syndrome (PNAS) or neonatal abstinence syndrome (NAS) if the mother has been on an antidepressant during pregnancy (especially an SSRI or SNRI). This reflects serotonin toxicity or overstimulation. The symptoms in the newborn are distress, fussiness, being jittery, abnormal crying, underactivity and difficulty feeding in the first few days of life. Such symptoms usually resolve in days or weeks but can last up to six weeks.
- The older antidepressants, the tricyclics (TCAs), are considered to confer only a slightly increased risk of foetal abnormalities. Despite their safety over many decades, instead of them the SSRIs are recommended in most current guidelines as the first-line antidepressant medication.

THE BENEFITS OF TREATING DEPRESSION DURING PREGNANCY

A review of the scientific literature[4] indicated that leaving depression untreated during pregnancy may delay body and head growth in the foetus, contribute to a lower body weight at birth, and be associated with increased behavioural difficulties (such as irritability, decreased activity) and greater developmental delay. Interpretation of such data is limited due to small sample sizes and relevant data often not having been recorded.

The following valuable guidelines are adapted from a published review.[5]

General strategies for antidepressant use during pregnancy

- Monotherapy (that is, only one medication) is best if possible and at the lowest effective dose, and medication should not be ceased abruptly.

- Where possible, exposure to antidepressants or antidepressants in combination with an existing benzodiazepine should be avoided during the first trimester.
- If the depression is severe, it is best to continue antidepressants; tapering and discontinuing before delivery risks recurrence of depression after the birth.

RESOURCES AND FURTHER READING
- beyondblue: www.beyondblue.org.au
- Motherisk (Canada): www.motherisk.org/women/index.jsp
- MotherSafe (Australia): www.mothersafe.org.au; helpline: 1800 647 848
- Perinatal Psychotropic Medicine Information Service: www.ppmis.org.au; helpline: (03) 8345 3190

Glossary

Words in italics have their own definition in the glossary.

Affective disorder/illness: see *Mood disorder.*

Antipsychotic medication: Medication supplied to prevent or relieve a psychotic episode. Can also be used to settle a manic high or added to an antidepressant to augment its antidepressant action.

Anxiety: A free-floating feeling of worry, nervousness or unease. See also *Panic attack.*

Bipolar or bipolar disorder: Once called manic depressive illness. An affective disorder characterised by episodes of mania (highs) or *hypomania* alone, and with depressive episodes (lows and commonly melancholic episodes) at other times. It is now subdivided into *bipolar I* and *bipolar II.*

Bipolar I: Involves episodes of both *mania* and *depression.* The highs are more severe, last longer and are often associated with delusions and/or hallucinations.

Bipolar II: Involves episodes of both *hypomania* and *melancholic depression* (but no psychotic experiences).

Clinical depression: An episode of *depression* that is severe, persistent and impairing. Clinical intervention is often needed to reach *remission.*

Cognitive behavioural therapy (CBT): A technique that provides tools to help alleviate the negative mindset of *depression* by combating irrational self-judgements.

Counselling: Involves listening, empathy and helping the client make sense of their experience and find strategies to deal with their difficulties. It may be used alone or in combination with other treatment.

Delusional depression: Also termed psychotic depression. The sufferer experiences false beliefs (delusions) and/or false perceptions (hallucinations) during a depressive episode. *Puerperal psychosis* is an acute condition with a sudden onset occurring close to childbirth. It may be psychotic depression, maniac or mixed state.

Depression: A broad term that can mean normal mood states, clinical syndromes and disease states (such as *melancholia*). At the *clinical depression* level, it affects body, mood and thoughts, and colours the sufferers' view of themselves. It can range from mild to very severe (*psychosis*, suicidal thoughts) and the sufferer seems unable to bounce back to their typical mood state without clinical intervention.

Depressogenic event: A stressful life event (such as loss of job, serious family dispute) that is likely to cause or precipitate *depression*. In someone with *bipolar disorder*, stressful events can bring on *hypomania*.

Diurnal variation: A change in depressive mood and energy level at certain times of the day. Often those with *melancholic depression* report lower mood and energy in the morning, while those with *non-melancholic depression* describe the opposite, and those with *psychotic depression* report no diurnal variation.

ECT (electroconvulsive therapy): A treatment that is effective across a narrow range of psychiatric disorders. It is the most effective antidepressant treatment for *melancholia* and *delusional depression* if other treatments have been unsuccessful, but is avoided up to that point because of its *side effects* (some impact on memory) and community unease (though surveys of those who have had ECT treatment endorse it as effective and acceptable).

General practitioner (GP): A medical doctor who provides primary care. A GP treats acute (short-term) and chronic (long-term) illnesses, and provides preventive care and health education for all age groups. Many embrace management of *mood disorders*.

High: The abnormal upswing in mood that is characteristic of *hypomania* or *mania*.

HPA axis: The hypothalamic–pituitary–adrenal axis is the body's mechanism for regulating systems such as temperature, digestion, immune system, mood, sexuality and energy usage. It also controls reaction to stress, trauma and injury. It is highly likely to be poorly regulated during episodes of *melancholia*. The challenges of the perinatal period can provide disruptions to HPA regulation.

Hypervigilance: An anxiety state of being too switched-on. The sufferer is abnormally watchful and on guard, scanning their surroundings for threats, easily startled and overreactive.

Hypomania: A *high* that is less extreme than the highs of a manic episode, and without any psychotic features.

Labile mood: Changeable, unsteady, easily altered emotions.

Major depression: A DSM (*Diagnostic and Statistical Manual of Mental Disorders*) diagnosis describing an episode of *depression* with five or more specific features (such as depressed mood, loss of interest and pleasure, sleep disturbance) that are present for two weeks or more and associated with social impairment.

Mania: A high mood of distinct severity where the sufferer is psychotic and experiences delusions and/or hallucinations.

Melancholia/melancholic depression: A biological subtype of *depression* that is genetically caused and impacts via creating a chemical imbalance in brain neurotransmitters, and which is more likely to start without any clearly explanatory *stressors*. It responds preferentially to physical (rather than psychological) treatments, such as antidepressant medication. Its clinical features can include slowed movement and a non-reactive mood.

Mood disorder (or affective disorder): A mental health problem characterised by distortion of mood—the profound sadness or apathy of *depression*, the euphoria and *highs* of *bipolar disorder*, or swings from one to the other.

Panic attack: An acute episode of *anxiety* where the sufferer experiences a racing heart, dizziness, headaches, or other physical symptoms. It is so severe and physical that sufferers may believe they are, for instance, about to die or have a stroke or are going mad.

Perinatal: In this book, the time from the start of pregnancy to the end of the baby's first year.

Perinatal depression: A depressive episode that occurs during the *perinatal* period.

Physical treatment: A treatment (such as antidepressant medication or ECT) designed to modify biological processes as opposed to psychological interventions that focus on the intra-psychic (mental) world of the individual.

Postnatal depression (PND): Any type of depression in a mother during the first 12 months after the birth of her baby.

Postpartum: Occurring after childbirth.

Postpartum psychosis: See *Puerperal psychosis*.

Primary and secondary conditions: The word 'primary' as in 'primary depression' indicates that the condition stands alone. 'Secondary depression' generally indicates that the *depression* follows, or is related to, another major medical condition, whether psychiatric (such as an *anxiety* disorder), medical (such as a stroke) or another factor (such as alcohol abuse).

Prophylactic medication: Medication prescribed to prevent a disorder from occurring or recurring, even when the disorder is not currently active.

Proximal and distal stressors: Proximal *stressors* (those in the sufferer's recent and/or current life) and distal *stressors* (those in the sufferer's past) are provided by situations and environments the sufferer experiences as unpleasant, and cause strain that can distort their development.

Psychogenic psychosis: An acute *psychosis* in predisposed individuals that occurs in reaction to stress. It tends to pass within days or weeks.

Psychosis: An impairment of mental functioning in which the sufferer loses touch with reality, experiencing delusions and/or hallucinations.

Psychotherapy: A non-physical treatment in which a therapist adopts a particular structure (such as analytic, interpersonal, cognitive, *cognitive behavioural therapy* techniques) to address symptoms and/or personality problems. A number of non-specific components, such as empathy, also make a therapeutic contribution.

Psychotic depression: See *Delusional depression*.

Psychotropic medication: Medication capable of affecting the mind, emotions and behaviour and used in the treatment of psychiatric disorders such as *depression, bipolar disorder* and *anxiety*.

Puerperal psychosis: A serious disorder in which a new mother loses touch with reality, becomes disoriented and may have hallucinations and disturbed delusions about herself, the baby and others, and experience rapid mood swings.

Recovery: When a depressive episode has completely resolved for a defined period.

Recurrence: A new episode of the same condition—a further instance of a bipolar *high*, for instance, is known as a recurrence of the disorder.

Relapse: The return of an episode of *depression* when the sufferer has not completely recovered from an earlier episode.

Remission: When a condition improves—but only for a brief period before recurring.

Resolve: (of symptoms) Disappear or dissipate.

Risk factors: A vulnerability that increases the possibility of developing a particular condition or disease. Examples include age, genetics, situations such as traumatic events, or the physical or psychological environment.

Rumination: A process of continually mulling over or brooding on negative experiences: problem-solving gone awry. It is repetitive, circular and disabling, but psychological techniques can arrest it.

Self-esteem: Also known as self-worth or self-regard. How we generally view ourselves. If positive, we regard ourselves as worthwhile and valuable; if negative, as worthless and useless. Historically, low self-esteem was called an 'inferiority complex'. *Depression* is partially defined as a drop in the individual's base levels of self-esteem.

Side effects: Unintended effects of medication that can exist alongside any positive effects of the medication, usually most pronounced during the first few weeks of treatment, but may appear after a time (such as weight gain, thyroid dysfunction).

Somatic: To do with the body, for example, a somatic (physical) illness. Sometimes depression or anxiety disorder may manifest as physical symptoms for which no underlying cause can be found.

Stigma: A sense of shame felt by people, particularly those with mental illness or other disability, as they attempt to function in the face of discrimination from the community.

Stressor: An event or interpersonal interaction that causes distress. Stressors can be acute (short-term, such as the immediate aftermath of an accident) or chronic (ongoing, such as poverty, a poor marriage). See also *Proximal and distal stressors*.

Syndrome: Signs and symptoms that occur together in a particular condition or illness.

Trait: An ongoing feature, such as personality style, underpinned by genetics.

Notes

Chapter 1: What are perinatal mood disorders?

1 E. Tom, 'Up the duff wouldn't be so rough but for the natal Nazis', *The Australian*, 30 July 2009.

2 Australian Institute of Health and Welfare, Metadata Online Registry, meteor.aihw.gov.au/content/index.phtml/itemId/327314, accessed April 2013.

3 Black Dog Institute Depression Education Program, 'DepEd: a guide to understanding and managing depression', www.blackdoginstitute. org.au/public/depression/depressioneducationprogram.cfm.

4 G. Parker and V. Manicavasagar, *Modelling and Managing the Depressive Disorders: A Clinical Guide*, Cambridge University Press, New York, 2005.

5 B. Shields, *Down Came the Rain: A Mother's Story of Postnatal Depression*, Penguin, Melbourne, 2005.

6 H. Murkoff, A. Eisenberg and S. Hathaway, 'Postpartum: the first six weeks', Chapter 16 in *What to Expect When You're Expecting*, 3rd edn, HarperCollins, Sydney, 2003, p. 405.

7 M.W. O'Hara and A.M. Swain, 'Rates and risk of postpartum depression: a meta-analysis', *International Review of Psychiatry*, vol. 8, no. 1, 1996, pp. 37–54.

8 P. Boyce, J. Condon, J. Barton and C. Corkindale, 'First-Time Fathers Study: psychological distress in expectant fathers during pregnancy', *Australian and New Zealand Journal of Psychiatry*, vol. 41, 2007, pp. 718–25.

9 P. Boyce and E. Barriball, 'Puerperal psychosis', *Archives of Women's Mental Health*, vol. 13, 2010, pp. 45–7.

10 T. Munk-Olsen, T.M. Laursen, S. Meltzer-Brody, P.B. Mortensen and
I. Jones, 'Psychiatric disorders with postpartum onset: possible early
manifestations of bipolar affective disorders', *Archives of General
Psychiatry*, vol. 69, 2012, pp. 428–34.

11 Black Dog Institute, 'Bipolar disorder explained', www.blackdog
institute.org.au/public/bipolardisorder/bipolardisorderexplained/
index.cfm.

12 G. Parker (ed.), *Bipolar II Disorder: Modelling, Measuring and
Managing*, Cambridge University Press, Cambridge, 2012.

13 Black Dog Institute, 'Self-test for depression during pregnancy and postnatally', www.blackdoginstitute.org.au/docs/Self-testingfordepression
inpregnancyandthepostnatalperiod.pdf; 'Self-test for bipolar disorder',
www.blackdoginstitute.org.au/public/bipolardisorder/self-test.cfm.

Chapter 2: Risk factors for perinatal mood problems

1 P. Boyce and A. Hickey, 'Psychosocial risk factors to major depression after childbirth', *Social Psychiatry and Psychiatric Epidemiology*,
vol. 40, 2005, pp. 605–12.

2 The 13HEALTH number (13 432 584) is a Queensland-only service.
The national Healthdirect service is available 24 hours a day, seven
days a week: call 1800 022 222 to talk to a registered nurse.

3 NSW Multicultural Health Communication Service (MHCS), www.
mhcs.health.nsw.gov.au; Transcultural Mental Health Centre, www.
dhi.health.nsw.gov.au/tmhc/default.aspx.

4 Down Syndrome Victoria, www.dsav.asn.au; for similar organisations
in other states, see www.downsyndrome.org.au.

Chapter 3: Screening for perinatal depression

1 C.A. Chew-Graham, D. Sharp, E. Chamberlain, L. Folkes and K.M.
Turner, 'Disclosure of symptoms of postnatal depression, the perspectives of health professionals and women: a qualitative study', *BioMed
Central Family Practice*, vol. 10, p. 7, 2009, www.biomedcentral.
com/1471-2296/10/7.

2 beyondblue, 'A guide to emotional health and wellbeing during pregnancy and early parenthood', www.bspg.com.au/dam/bsg/product?
client=BEYONDBLUE&prodid=BL/0943&type=file; 'Managing mental
health conditions during pregnancy and early parenthood: a
guide for women and their families', www.bspg.com.au/dam/bsg/

product?client=BEYONDBLUE&prodid=BL/0944&type=file; see also
www.beyondblue.org.au/the-facts/pregnancy-and-early-parenthood.

3 M.A. Whooley, A.L. Avins, J. Miranda and W.S. Browner, 'Case-
   finding instruments for depression: two questions are as good
   as many', *Journal of General Internal Medicine*, vol. 12, 1997,
   pp. 439–45.
4 D. Gjerdingen, S. Crow, P. McGovern, M. Miner and B. Center,
   'Postpartum depression screening at well-child visits: validity of a
   2-question screen and the PHQ–9', *Annals of Family Medicine*, vol. 7,
   2009, pp. 63–70.
5 D. Goyal, C. Gay and K. Lee, 'Fragmented maternal sleep is more
   strongly correlated with depressive symptoms than infant temperament at three months postpartum', *Archives of Women's Mental
   Health*, vol. 12, 2009, pp. 229–37.
6 M-P. Austin, J. Colton, S. Priest, N. Reilly and D. Hadzi-Pavlovic,
   'The antenatal risk questionnaire (ANRQ): acceptability and use for
   psychosocial risk assessment in the maternity setting', *Women and
   Birth*, vol. 26, 2013, pp. 17–25.
7 J.L. Cox, J.M. Holden and R. Sagovsky, 'Detection of postnatal depression. Development of the 10-item Edinburgh Postnatal Depression
   Scale', *British Journal of Psychiatry*, vol. 150, 1987, pp. 782–6.
8 A. López, 'Perinatal depression: early detection, prevention and treatment', Wild Iris Medical Education, Inc., 2010, www.nursingceu.com/
   courses/279/index_nceu.html.
9 Black Dog Institute professional education training course, 'Perinatal
   mood disorders in practice'.
10 Families NSW, 'Improving mental health outcomes for parents and
   infants: SAFE START guidelines', 2009, www.sfe.nswiop.nsw.edu.au/
   file.php/1/SafeStartGuidelines.pdf.

Chapter 4: Diagnosis and treatment options

1 G. Parker, A. Paterson, K. Fletcher, M. Hyett and B. Blanch, 'Out of
   the darkness: the impact of a mood disorder over time', *Australasian
   Psychiatry*, vol. 20, 2012, pp. 487–91.
2 Black Dog Institute professional education training course, 'Perinatal
   mood disorders in practice'.

Chapter 5: Protecting yourself with realistic expectations

1 M. Freedman, 'A pain in the guts', Life Matters, Sunday Life, *Sun-Herald*, 16 May 2011, p. 9.

2 J.L. Barkin and K.L. Wisner, 'The role of maternal self-care in new motherhood', *Midwifery*, 29 (9), pp. 1050–5.

Chapter 6: Learning to live in Motherland

1 E. Bombeck, *Motherhood: The Second Oldest Profession*, Futura, London, 1984.

2 V. Gordon, Black Dog Institute General Practice Education Program Developer.

3 J. Evans, J. Heron, H. Francomb, S. Oke and J. Golding, 'Cohort study of depressed mood during pregnancy and after childbirth', *British Medical Journal*, vol. 323, 2001, pp. 257–60.

4 K.A. Yonkers, M.V. Smith, N. Gotman and K. Belanger, 'Typical somatic symptoms of pregnancy and their impact on a diagnosis of major depressive disorder', *General Hospital Psychiatry*, vol. 31, 2009, pp. 327–33.

5 N. Edwards, P.G. Middleton, D.M. Blyton and C.E. Sullivan, 'Sleep disordered breathing and pregnancy', *Thorax*, vol. 57, 2002, pp. 555–8.

6 H. Chilton, 'A quick "set-up guide" to your new baby', Chapter 1 in H. Chilton, *Baby on Board: Understanding Your Baby's Needs in the First Twelve Months*, 2nd edn, Finch Publishing, Sydney, 2009, pp. 2, 3; www.babycentre.co.uk/x553877/how-do-i-know-if-my-baby-latched-on-correctly, accessed March 2013.

7 D. Goyal, C. Gay and K. Lee, 'Fragmented maternal sleep is more strongly correlated with depressive symptoms than infant temperament at three months postpartum', *Archives of Women's Mental Health*, vol. 12, 2009, pp. 229–37.

8 H. Hiscock and M. Wake, 'Infant sleep problems and post-natal depression: a community-based study', *Pediatrics*, vol. 107, 2001, pp. 1317–22.

9 R. Cusk, 'Motherbaby', Section 6 in *A Life's Work: On Becoming a Mother*, Fourth Estate, London, 2001, pp. 104, 105.

10 H. Chilton, 'Colic and the unsettled baby', Chapter 15 in Chilton, *Baby on Board*, pp. 180–91.

Chapter 7: Do you need help?

1 G. Greenberg, *Manufacturing Depression*, Bloomsbury, London, 2010, p. 367

2 Black Dog Institute, 'Self-test for bipolar disorder', www.blackdog institute.org.au/public/bipolardisordcr/self-test.cfm.

3 beyondblue, 'Barriers for women and their families', Section 1.4, Subsection 1.4.1 in *Clinical Practice Guidelines: Depression and Related Disorders—Anxiety, Bipolar Disorder and Puerperal Psychosis—in the Perinatal Period: A Guideline for Primary Care Health Professionals*, February 2011, p. 5, www.beyondblue.org.au/resources/ health-professionals/clinical-practice-guidelines/perinatal-clinical-practice-guidelines.

Chapter 8: Where to get help

1 Boyce and Hickey, 'Psychosocial risk factors to major depression after childbirth'.

Chapter 9: Tackling stigma and mothers' guilt

1 F. Bacon, 'Of parents and children', *The Essays*, Penguin, London, 1985, p. 79.

2 N. Ghaemi, 'Stigma and politics', Chapter 15 in N. Ghaemi, *A First-rate Madness: Uncovering the Links between Leadership and Mental Illness*, Penguin, New York, 2011, pp. 256–65.

3 Gordon W. Allport, *The Nature of Prejudice*, Perseus, New York, 1979 (first published 1954), p. xvii.

4 J. Masserman, 'Faith and delusion in psychotherapy: the ur-defenses of man', *American Journal of Psychiatry*, vol. 110, 1953, pp. 324–33.

5 Barkin and Wisner, 'The role of maternal self-care in new motherhood'.

6 C.C. Weitzman and Yale Medical Group, 'Beyond postpartum: treating depression in mothers of older children', Pediatric Academic Societies Annual Meeting, Vancouver, Canada, 1 May 2010.

7 D. Quinton, M. Rutter and C. Liddle, 'Institutional rearing, parental difficulties and marital support', *Psychological Medicine*, vol. 14, 1984, pp. 107–24.

8 G. Parker and D. Hadzi-Pavlovic, 'Modification of levels of depression in mother-bereaved women by parental and marital relationships', *Psychological Medicine*, vol. 14, 1984, pp. 125–35.

9   L. Kilmartin, K. Moline, A. Ybarbo and M. Zoeller, *Sh*tty Mom: The Parenting Guide for the Rest of Us*, Abrams, New York, 2012, p. 168.
10   E. Wilson, 'Motherhood, mind and body', *Times Literary Supplement*, 16 November 2012, p. 5.
11   Bombeck, *Motherhood*.
12   G. Parker, A. Paterson, K. Fletcher, B. Blanch and R. Graham, 'The "magic button question" for those with a mood disorder—would they wish to re-live their condition?' *Journal of Affective Disorders*, vol. 136, 2012, pp. 419–24.

Chapter 10: Managing a mood disorder and maintaining recovery

1   MotherSafe, local advisory centres, www.seslhd.health.nsw.gov.au/mothersafe/Local.asp.
2   S. Mares, L. Newman, B. Warren and K. Cornish, *Clinical Skills in Infant Mental Health*, ACER Press, Melbourne, 2005.
3   Kilmartin, Moline, Ybarbo and Zoeller, *Sh*tty Mom*, p. 162.
4   A. Buist, 'Treatment of perinatal depression', *Australian Prescriber*, vol. 31, 2008, pp. 36–9; M-P. Austin and S.R. Priest, 'Clinical issues in perinatal mental health: new developments in the detection and treatment of perinatal mood and anxiety disorders', *Acta Psychiatrica Scandinavica*, vol. 112, 2005, pp. 97–104.

Chapter 11: Fathers and the extended family

1   M. and A. Johnstone, *Living with a Black Dog*, Pan Macmillan, Sydney, 2008.

Appendix: Medications in the perinatal period

1   L.H. Chaudron, 'Complex challenges in treating depression during pregnancy', *American Journal of Psychiatry*, vol. 170, 2013, pp. 12–20.
2   N. Byatt, K.M. Deligiannidis and M.P. Freeman, 'Antidepressant use in pregnancy: a critical review focused on risks and controversies', *Acta Psychiatrica Scandinavica*, vol. 127, 2013, pp. 94–114.
3   M.A. De Vera and A. Bérard, 'Antidepressant use during pregnancy and the risk of pregnancy-induced hypertension', *British Journal of Clinical Pharmacology*, vol. 74, 2012, pp. 362–9.
4   Chaudron, 'Complex challenges in treating depression during pregnancy'.
5   Chaudron, 'Complex challenges in treating depression during pregnancy'.

Index

abortion, unwanted 50–2
advice 109–10
affective disorder 221
agitation 17, 24
Allport, Gordon 154
anergia 17
anger 13, 17, 54, 83, 130, 133, 176
anhedonia 19
another baby, decision to have 183–4
antenatal risk questionnaire (ANRQ), 67
antipsychotic medication 219
  pregnancy and 214
anxiety 1, 14, 15, 113, 123, 155, 170, 171
  definition 219
  depression and 14, 143
  panic attacks 15, 41, 117, 130, 173, 221
  postnatal anxiety group 178
  postnatal depression and 21, 123
  risk factors 40–4
  stressors 16
assessment *see also* diagnosis; screening
  background information 143
  content 143
  family deciding if needed 199–200
  health professional, by 80–4
  risk assessment 143, 144
  what to expect 144
Australian Breastfeeding Association 138, 142

baby
  bonding with 159–61
  crying 42, 54–5, 77, 80–3, 109–10, 129–30, 176, 201
  decision to have another 183–4
  difficult 117–118, 143, 170
  failure to bond with 6, 7–10, 18, 113
  father's interaction with 92
  fear of harm to 25, 130, 131, 144, 157–8
  fear that baby will be taken away 79–80, 122
  frustration and anger with 83, 130
  inability to care for 21, 118, 177
  infanticide 24
  preoccupation with health of 24, 130, 171
  resentment of 93, 133
  risk of harm to 23, 24, 144
  sleep 107–9, 138, 202
  temperament of 49, 54
  thoughts of harming 121, 130, 137, 143, 144, 176, 177